A WORM IN THE TEACHER'S APPLE

PROTECTING AMERICA'S SCHOOL CHILDREN FROM PESTS AND PESTICIDES

by
MARC L. LAME

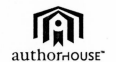

authorHOUSE™

1663 LIBERTY DRIVE, SUITE 200
BLOOMINGTON, INDIANA 47403
(800) 839-8640
WWW.AUTHORHOUSE.COM

First published by AuthorHouse 05/04/05

ISBN: 1-4208-3935-7 (sc)

Library of Congress Control Number: 2005903546

Printed in the United States of America
Bloomington, Indiana

This book is printed on acid-free paper.

This book is dedicated to my daughters Samantha and Shannon. They sacrificed their time with "Dad" so that I might help more daughters and sons. They teach me everyday, and, just so they know, "it is all about you".

Preface

Some parents and many school officials are aware that there is a substantial movement to create a safer learning environment in our nation's schools. Not just in terms of violent acts, but in terms of environmental quality. Over 30 states have legislation requiring schools to reduce the unnecessary exposure of children to pesticides. These mandates range from having plans on site explaining the best management practices for pest management, to designating a district pest management coordinator, to notifying parents and teachers prior to the application of pesticides. I decided to write this book because, with very few exceptions, school districts throughout the nation (whether in these 30 states or not) are not implementing cost effective pest management so as to minimize the problems of pests and pesticides. As with so many other mandates, promises, and intentions, our decision makers at the local, state and federal levels of education and children's health protection seem satisfied that regulations, policies, plans and manuals are solving the problem. Sure, these are critical parts of the solution, but it doesn't occur unless someone actually does it – rather than talks about it, legislates it, or has it on the shelf. Pest management is people management. We know that school officials have enough to worry about already – budget cuts, testing, the threat of becoming another Columbine High School and terrorism.

The fact is that our schools are using our tax monies to apply sometimes dangerous chemicals where our children learn. That wouldn't be so bad if these applications were preventing the diseases attributed to pests, harmful bites and stings and the nuisance of "bugs" in the classroom. However, in most cases schools are paying for traditional pest control strategies which result in substandard pest reduction and, indeed, often an increase in the spread of pest populations throughout the school. Go figure - more money, more pesticides, and more pests and all this, when our children need fewer pesticides, fewer pests and more effective spending for education.

I am an entomologist and a parent. I am not going to sit here and write that chemical pesticides are bad and should be eliminated. Fact is, Rachel Carson in *Silent Spring* did not say that either. What you will read in both of our books (my clever way of linking this measly text to that of my hero) is that pesticides should not be used unnecessarily. The environment doesn't deserve it and sure as hell my twin daughters don't. Like most parents, I want to know what is going on in my kids' lives. I want to know what is making them happy or sad, what is stimulating them to learn, or what/who is inhibiting the development of my children's intellect.

I want to know that institutions I trust are protecting my kids, and if not, why? When my babies went off to kindergarten their first day, didn't I walk them into the room and give the teacher my best "your life depends on these girls coming home safe, happy, and smart" glare? On their second day, didn't my wife and I discuss dressing in camouflage and following them to school? And, didn't I feel sick to my stomach watching the anguish of the Columbine High School children and parents? My point is I do not expose my children to unnecessary risks.

The material in this book is intended for teachers, school officials, regulators, parents and pest management professionals. While it includes scientific information, it deals with people management and communication problems with solutions that will provide a safe learning environment in terms of pests—mostly insect pests. I can write scientific articles for "peer reviewed" journals, but I want to write this book to be one that real people can read and understand. I don't need tenure and who reads "peer reviewed" journals anyway? It is my hope, that by telling the story of how schools address their real or perceived pests, those of you participating in the school community can become aware of the problems, solutions, and "stonewalling" that impact our children's health.

This book will anger some people, but it is what it is. If I have learned anything during my 20-plus years as an entomologist, environmental regulator, and childcare advocate, it is that institutions are slow to change. It takes a crisis. AND, it takes activists to point out the crisis and the need for solutions. This book begs for those activists (parents and educators) and I hope it provides the solution for a safer learning environment for our children.

Acknowledgements

There is no way I can feel the pain of childbirth, but I now have vastly more sympathy for a mother who is even one week overdue delivering her baby. Originally I thought writing this book would take about one year. Four years later I just want it OUT! However, I did want the process of writing and publishing this book to result in a healthy, beautiful, bouncing and happy product.

Bill Norman, my old friend who stood back-to-back with me during my days at the Arizona Department of Environmental Quality, edited this book. He called it *The Thing* and *Monster* as we corresponded by e-mail. I can't thank you enough. Though, imagine what it would have looked like if Tom Neltner, Rebecca Schmitt and Carl Martin had not proof read it first? Stacy Elko is the incredible artist who illustrated the cover of this book, and January Jones nearly wore out her camera trying to come up with a picture of me for the back cover. Both women are tolerant to a fault. To my friends, colleagues and family I will always be grateful for your support:

Fred Whitford at Purdue University told me in 1995 that if I did not intend on publishing on our efforts it would be a waste of time. As we have visited over the years, there has not been a time when he hasn't reminded me to publish. Okay Fred, I have followed your advice, but be careful what you wished for because this book will not please many in our profession.

There is no way I could have learned enough and/or sustained my efforts without my teammates. You all are providing the "truth" for this book everyday. My special "Bloomington Homeboys" - Jerry Jochim and John Carter who believed I really knew what I was talking about and provided me with a sympathetic ear, beer and bad food when the going got tough. Mike Lindsey and Carl Olson, who dearly love to watch me fight the good fight. Carl Martin, Lyn Hawkins, Stan Peterson, Jennifer Snyder, Roy Morris, David Peterson, Faith Oi, Rebecca Baldwin, Norm Leppla, Earl Lewallen, Richard Smith, Mike Ward, Allen Wilson, Larry Pinto, Richard Lumpkin and Fudd Graham who reposed faith in me to learn when in fact, they were teaching. Bobby Corrigan, my urban pest management mentor, friend and reluctant travel companion, whose calm, patient ways allowed me to learn and his unflagging defense of our planet and profession demonstrated to me he is a man of honor. Dawn Gouge, not just my teammate but my partner in changing the world. More than anyone, Dawn had a way of letting me believe I could publish this book – that it was supremely important. Fly free Tonbo.

There are former and current employees of the USEPA who, not only made sure I was giving the taxpayers their monies worth, but provided guidance, direction and encouragement during the development and implementation of the Monroe IPM Model. Further, they insisted that I write the process down so others might use it. Jim Boland, Ralph Wright and Bill Curry (all retired); Sherry Glick, Kathy Seikel, Debra Hartman, Darlene Dinkins, Mary Grisier, Don Baumgartner, Troy Pierce and Janet Andersen who always maintained the highest of standards. Most important, these professionals believe in Integrated Pest Management and care about your children.

Tom Green, Mike Wallace, Jay Feldman and Tom Neltner - The not-for-profit organization advocates for Integrated Pest Management and children's environmental health who enlightened me to the needs of the public and how Integrated Pest Management should be used. Max Bass, Jim Harper, Gary Mullen and Mike Williams – my professors at Auburn University who opened the door for me to become an entomologist, and Chuck Triplehorn at Ohio State University who treated me like an entomologist before I was one. Thank-you Al Greene, for trying to teach us all that we should "do IPM because it is the right thing for our children", (and letting me paraphrase you). Thanks, Leon Moore and Theo Watson, for making me your "pitbull", teaching me when to get off the fence and that "you aren't working if your hands aren't dirty".

I could not be a professional educator without students. They say "the best way to learn is to teach". David Hokanson, Linda Debrewer, Terry Babcock-Lumish, Kristi Kubista-Hovis, January Jones and Rebecca Schmitt contributed to this book as scholars, reviewers and photographers. However, I wish to thank them more so for allowing me to learn while teaching them. And I thank my campers and counselors at Camp Roosevelt for attending my Nature Hikes so that I could be among the trees and watch the bees.

Ed Fox and Jim Barnes are my former bosses and honorable men who allowed me to learn to become a public official who must respect our citizens; understand that environmental professionals have an obligation to work with the USEPA; and recognize environmental law for the double-edged sword that it is. Yes, Ed, I am having fun.

My late father, Dr. Louis A. Lame, came home from the horrors of war to become a pediatrician. He wanted me to help others with "the laying on of hands" – I acknowledge your wish and wisdom. My mother, Pauli K. Lame always encouraged my love of nature. Her uncompromising ethics brought me to this book.

My incredible wife, Chriss, and daughters, Samantha and Shannon, have a husband and father who is an entomologist and environmentalist. Yet, you tolerated me and supported my need to write this book. I am sorry about keeping collected insects in our freezer – I should have told you they weren't chocolate chips.

In memoriam, thank you, Everett Rogers, for *Diffusion of Innovations* and for enjoying teaching an entomologist that IPM was something people must adopt; Kent Samsel for believing in the particular brand of humor to which I so shamelessly subject my readers to; President Theodore Roosevelt's role model for naturalists who want to change the world and to Rachel Carson for changing the world with *Silent Spring*.

Finally, I acknowledge the Trees, Stars and the Moon. Mokuso – I am ready.

Contents

PART I:
Problems

Chapter One – There is no "Silver Bullet" but there is a "Treadmill"

When I was nine years old exploring the world, I attended Camp Wing-a-Roo in Perry, Ohio. I was a "nature boy". I would work very hard to be Mickey Mantle in right field only to find myself staring at a spider eating a fly atop the dandelion. Inevitably, a ball would head out my way and I would miss it — no wonder I always played right field. But, I didn't miss how the spider was almost invisible to both me and the fly, and how everything about it seemed built for catching bugs. I would sneak away from tennis (like I could *play* tennis) to the patch of milkweed next to the courts and catch honey bees – with my bare hands. Neat trick, pinching both sets of wings together behind their back as they gathered pollen. They couldn't sting me – too often. Or, during our swimming lessons I would study the water boatman swimming just below the surface of the pool and wonder: "If its legs look like oars, how could it walk into the pool"?

I could go on. I have *lots* of memories of bugs as a kid. People often ask me, "What made you decide to become an entomologist"? The answer is easy — I was that kind of kid. You know what I mean. A lot of you might have kids like me (sorry, mom). Rest assured most grow out of the bug watching, catching, eating stage. Not me. That's not to say that from age 13 to 26 my hormones didn't overcome my fascination with bugs. As a student at Ohio State University, trying to get into veterinary school, I was given the choice of taking advanced calculus or entomology to fulfill my undergrad requirements. Calculus? During that first entomology class I realized that one could make a living playing with bugs. Vet school wasn't going to happen anyway.

"Silver Bullets" – Better Living Through Chemistry

In 1961 I was a 9-year-old kid at that same summer camp in northeastern Ohio. I found myself playing in a sweet smelling fog (most likely DDT), which hours later was responsible for fish floating in the creek in which I spent so many hours being a "nature boy". There was an orchard next to the camp and when the spray rig wafted through, we all loved to play in the fog. Of course, I couldn't connect the significance of the two situations at the age of nine. Worse yet, neither could my adult caretakers. For them the "silver bullet" of pesticides had no collateral damage.

Seven years later, as a counselor in training, I had the really cool duty of mosquito control (camp directors understandably were reluctant to let me teach baseball). I had a very temperamental fogger (it resembled a machine gun with an oversized barrel) which once humming could smoke out (fumigate) a cabin or campfire area in nothing flat. I felt like Sgt. Rock with this machine on my hip, doling out death to bugs. I would pour a few glugs (as in glug, glug — still a common measurement of pesticide mixtures) into the tank and let 'er rip. Walking through the fog — cool. I was very popular right before overnights and campfires.

"Silver Bullet" is a term that ecologist David Pimentel uses to describe what our culture really loves about science solving our problems. Whereas "silver bullets" may work well against werewolves and other fictional beasties, objective disease and pest managers know that the quick fix, while quite attractive, often doesn't work. Let's talk American agriculture, where two thirds of pesticides are used — through the same marketing strategies, from the same manufacturers and under the same federal regulatory agencies that apply to the pesticides used in your schools, restaurants, parks and homes.

The facts are that, since the advent of widespread synthetic pesticides (e.g., DDT, Chlordane, Methyl/Ethyl Parathion, Malathion, Chlorpyrifos and the synthetic pyrethroids), use of them in the United States has increased by a factor of 10, while damage from pests has doubled (Pimentel, 1997). I would bet that public health officials can provide similar statistics for antibiotics in relation to bacterial disease management.

Rachel Carson published *Silent Spring* in 1962. Her text changed the history of environmental management by exposing the overuse of pesticides in America, and she is my hero. At that time U.S. agriculture was using approximately 500 million pounds of pesticides annually to control pests in agriculture. Later, *The Pesticide Conspiracy*, by Robert Van Den Bosch (1978), had an even greater effect on the entomological establishment than *Silent Spring*. Van Den Bosch, an entomology professor at the University of California at Riverside, documented that insecticides were being used unnecessarily by farmers in the Southwest, causing health problems for both farm workers and certain animal populations (Van Den Bosch, 1978). Since these early books began creating an awareness of pesticide problems among the public and the applied entomological community, there have been literally thousands of human health and environmental impact studies published concerning the harmful effects of pesticides.

But is the system really changing? In 1992, we were using 900 million pounds, and in 2000, 940 million pounds of pesticides. Two important points here:

1) Active Ingredients (A.I. - the actual poison versus the inert "carrier" ingredients) are the calculated poundage in this study. Advances in technology have decreased the active ingredients substantially (sometimes from pounds to fractions of an ounce). You figure, how many more applications or exposures actually resulted from the increased poundage? I figure at least a factor of four; and

2) these increases took place when new policies, laws and plans were put in place during "green administrations", and my profession was supposedly enlightened with regard to pesticide use, misuse and resistance.

Again, I am not saying that pesticides are evil. Indeed, we would not be able to enjoy the health and standard of living we have today if it were not for the contribution of pesticides. Worldwide, millions of lives have been saved through mosquito control programs using insecticides to kill populations of these vectors of Malaria, Denge Fever, and West Nile Virus just to name a few of the many arthropod-borne diseases that humans are subjected to. We could not grow affordable crops on the amount of land we currently use without using pesticides. Thus, this chemical technology we call pesticides has its place in our lifestyle. But, they also have adverse health effects on our health and the environment. They have "…increased risks for cancer, neurological disorders, and endocrine and immune system dysfunction; impaired surface and ground water; and harm fish and wildlife." (GAO-01-815, p. 1, 2001) The statistics are out there. Two red herrings of the school pest management argument masquerade in the questions, "Are pesticides toxic to us?" and "Is there a cheaper way to control pests?" I will discuss these side-tracking ploys arguments later, but for now I prefer to explore the reasons why this conflict exists. Ultimately I will address the issue of how we can balance our lifestyles and environmental quality when it comes to pest management.

Are Insecticides Used Efficiently?

This question addresses the fundamental issue of insecticides as viewed in the context of management. Rather than presenting a long list of complex facts and figures related to insecticide use, misuse or reduction, one must specifically ask: "Given fiscal, environmental, and sociological constrains in any pest management situation, is the use and amount of pesticides absolutely necessary?" A more specific question could be: "If using a pesticide is the most effective tool to manage a pest situation, is the amount of material used the lowest possible?" This question almost always receives a resounding Yes! answer from users of pesticides. "After all, (they claim) using pesticides is costly—why would we ever use more than we absolutely had to?" In fact, the answer depends on what management system one is using.

Traditionally, the pesticide option and amount used have resulted from decisional guidelines determined by the government, bank, university Cooperative Extension, exterminator and chemical company. However, these guidelines were developed in response to policies which contradict the concept of modern pest management philosophy – that of "optimizing control rather than maximizing it" (Metcalf & Luckmann, p. 4, Basso, 1987). Here it would be instructive to understand what policy has to do with a management program.

This is called the planning process. A policy is a statement of goals and their relative import, which are then given specific objectives that transform the policy into a plan, which is implemented in the form of a program consisting of specific actions (Starling, 1993). So, the answer to the question, "Is the pesticide option and amount used warranted—as a specific program action to achieve a specific plan objective?" depends on the goals of the pest management policy.

National pest management policies in recent history have had the goals of maximizing control with the objectives of maximum yields, pest eradication and high cosmetic standards that required increased pesticide use as the specific actions of the management program (Basso, 1987). Thus, those professing that they use the least amount of pesticides to obtain the goals of traditional agricultural, structural and public health pest management programs are probably correct. But these goals are customer driven. What if we didn't need cosmetically perfect apples, or a sterile living/learning environment? If the goals of successful competition between humans and pests for food, fiber, shelter and attention were to optimize the control of pests through maximizing efficiency, there would be increased use of *rational* tools for pest management instead of "kill 'em all" with chemical pesticides.

How could this happen?

We don't need to use pesticides nearly as much as agrichemical companies (the folks that make and sell pesticides) tell us to— the same folks who tried to stop the New Yorker magazine from first publishing excerpts of Carson's book. A pest can be defined as an organism (insect, spider, rodent, reptile, plant, fungus, etc.) that competes with humans for food, water, shelter, or attention. The pests associated with the school environment seek out, utilize and inhabit the environment that the human population has created for the education of its children. Whereas *Heliothis zea* (cotton bollworm) competes with humans because a cultivated field represents their required habitat, *Musca domestica (*housefly) competes with humans because our habitat also represents their required habitat. Humans are fierce competitors. If we don't like it, and it competes with us, we want to kill it.

Agrichemical manufacturing and pest extermination companies spend lots of money to convince us that we should hate or, worse, fear all invaders. You have seen the commercials showing roaches and warning of diseases — spray inside; potbellied men whispering about the lethargic homeowner whose dandelion-infested yard is ruining the neighborhood – spray outside; ticks and mosquitoes sucking your blood and transmitting diseases - spray yourself! Did you ever ask yourself whose idea it was to have a perfectly green yard, red apple, or sterile house? Come on, admit it. Even if you do decide to buy those advertisements, and spray that nasty old roach, do you follow the label (it's the law!) and just give that six-legged monster one quick squirt? Horse pucky! You douse it! Scream at it! Drown it! And, if you don't have Raid® you use oven cleaner or hairspray. Hell, I know some of you (usually tough guys) have even used WD40® as a blow torch to incinerate it! Admit it. Entomologists love media stories about people burning down their houses this way. Even more fun are those who blow their houses up by overusing pesticide "bombs" in their airtight houses with the gas pilot light on. Bug humor.

We have been trained well through the manipulations of billions of dollars worth of advertising to be fierce competitors, and we have been given the weapons to succeed. How sexy is having "Robo-exterminator" patrolling the perimeter of your house to protect you? The agchem companies even have farmers believing that they are more patriotic if they use pesticides.

7

No kidding. Listen to the ads on early morning TV before planting season. To my great sadness (in that I spent more than 10 years working with the USDA to develop and extend less expensive and more environmentally sound pest management technology to farmers) it has been and still is their policy to promote the use of pesticides. It broke my heart when I found out that my agency, my government, also tried to prevent Rachel Carson from publishing her book. But, that's for later. There is a better way, and that is what most of this book is about.

In their text, *Introduction to Insect Pest Management* (first edition, 1975), Metcalf and Luckmann introduced several basic concepts which provided the foundation for a philosophy of rational pest management. This philosophy included discussions of why insects are pests: "... an insect becomes a pest because we call it one, and a pest problem exists because an insect is competing with man", and "Pest management concepts dictate a tolerant approach to pest status" (Metcalf and Luckmann, p. 2). They subscribed to Geier's (1966) description of the practice of pest management: knowing the numbers (determining economic thresholds); knowing the biology (manage to the vulnerabilities of the pest); and knowing the audience (knowing if the control program is acceptable-- environmentally, economically, and socially) by those implementing the control technologies.

Addressing the human aspect of pest management then reaches the point where pest management transforms itself from a biological/technical discipline to a sociological/management discipline whereby, "Insects can be managed, but management is people-oriented, and successful pest management depends largely on influencing the people who control the pest" (Metcalf and Luckmann, p. 2). If implementers (change agents) such as school district facility managers, university Cooperative Extension specialists and exterminators would plan programs that fit the school community's perceived risks and needs (as well as employ proper social and marketing/communication skills), proponents of rational pest control could successfully compete with people who sell and/or apply pesticides for a living (Wearing, 1988). Metcalf and Luckmann's 1975 prediction that the greatest obstacle to successful pest management is, in fact, the attitude of people. This remains our most formidable obstacle. Those who believe the "silver bullet" will solve our problems quickly and cheaply (customers, bureaucrats who hate change and/or fear upsetting the status quo, and those calling themselves professionals who find it more profitable to keep on spraying) do so based on an attitude that is opposed to more rational solutions.

8

Why aren't the "silver bullets" fixing our problems quickly and permanently? Two reasons: 1) Just as bullets are meant to kill the enemy (not prevent the aggression), the vast majority of pesticides are meant to kill the pest (not prevent the infestation); and 2) The enemy has bullet-proof vests — pests develop resistance to pesticides.

Up until the mid-twentieth century our ancestors planted crops knowing that one third would be eaten by species (we call them pests) other than us. They burned the crop trash or stubble before or after the season to destroy over-wintering pests and pest habitat. They would smoke meats and store them in a smoke house, keep grains in sealed containers, and yes, pick lice out of each others' hair (preening). And, we lived with a few bugs. Now we don't. We don't have to. We have pesticides – "better living through chemistry". And, I am damn' glad of it — particularly when it comes to lice. Unfortunately, we forgot everything else meaningful and have now become dependent on chemicals. We just douse pests or pay money to someone else who'll come to our homes, schools, restaurants and cotton fields once a month to kill them even more effectively.

Modern medical practitioners have learned that pharmaceuticals alone won't provide a better quality of life. We have to prevent poor health — exercise, eat better, smoke less More importantly, we must know what causes health problems, change our lifestyles to prevent problems and sometimes take the safest medicine in the most effective manner (remembering the current warnings to physicians not to over-prescribe antibiotics, and to patients, to "take as directed"). Just as with modern medicine, in managing pests we must learn what is causing the pest problem (we call that "conducive conditions" in the bug world), prevent an infestation by changing our behavior (e.g., plant to subvert the pests' lifecycle, clean our sinks, store our cereal in airtight containers, and yes, even become more tolerant of some pests) and use the safest pesticide in the most effective manner.

The idea that we or professional pesticide applicators can kill pests with even the safest pesticide doesn't by itself correct the problem any more than if we were to take a drug to lower blood pressure and continue to eat fatty foods and never exercise. What happens as soon as we quit taking the drug? We dare not, unless we have taken the other steps to allow our body to achieve lower blood pressure. What happens if our doctor continues to have us take antibiotics every time we go to her with a cold or we don't follow the directions regarding the effective use of that antibiotic? Over time, that behavior becomes ineffective.

Most living organisms have genetic defenses to protect them from deadly threats. There are always a few individuals in a population that are resistant to diseases, and over time (in our case, as humans, thousands of years) those resistant genes become part of the surviving population. With microbes it can be a matter of months or years. With insects, a matter of a few years — depending on how fast generations turn over and their degree of exposure to the antibiotic or insecticide (selective pressure). There you have it: my super short course on genetic resistance. More than 500 insect pests, 270 plant pests (weeds), and 150 diseases of plants are now resistant to one or more pesticides (GAO-01-815, 2001).

In his book *The Pesticide Conspiracy*, Robert Van Den Bosch describes the "Pesticide Treadmill". Simply put, when we became more dependent on pesticides as the advertised quick fix, insects, weeds and plant pathogens developed resistance at an increasing rate. Two things happened: 1) We had to apply more and more pesticides to control pest outbreaks for crop, structural or public health pests (thank you, Rachel Carson, for getting DDT banned in 1969, but the fact is that DDT really wasn't working on insects like tobacco budworms in cotton, mosquitoes in suburbs, or roaches in our houses anymore); and 2) Because most of our insecticides were and are broad spectrum (you've heard the advertisements that Kill-'em-all-let-God-sort-Them-Out® kills x, y, z bugs in your home and garden), they not only killed the non-resistant pestiferous insects, but also their natural predators and parasitoids — good bugs —the majority of species in fields and in and around our homes.

So let's get this straight. Over-reliance on chemical control produced "super bugs" AND killed off those other arthropods (insects, spiders and the like) that would normally keep them in check. Thus, we developed an expensive (in terms of damage and disease) and sometimes dangerous snowball effect of more applications, begetting more and stronger applications, begetting more and different applications...you get my drift.

Unless you are on top of the awareness scale and/or your school district is extremely progressive, I'd bet you don't know what your child's school (or you - if you are a teacher, custodian, kitchen, clerical or other staff working in a school) is doing to manage pests. Ask your school what it's doing to manage pests, *which* pests and with what technology? Is the person who applies pesticides licensed or is he/she a minimum waged technician working for someone who is? I will explain more of my rationale for these questions later, but I can tell you that the vast majority of school administrators (principals, facility managers, etc.) could not answer even *these* questions, let alone identify the hazards of either pests or pesticides. They just don't know. What you can probably bet is being done in your school is that once a month someone (licensed or not) is applying pesticides, usually on a Friday afternoon when the kids go home, somewhere on campus — whether it's needed or not. Of course there are many worse case scenarios — an insecticide is sprayed into the air ducts of your school by an uneducated applicator, five students are hospitalized, and the school gets evacuated. It happens more often than we can imagine. There is a better way.

Chapter Two – Back to School, Dr. Lame – The Reality of Agrichemicals

It all started with a very angry mother (I will call her Maude) who was a mighty pain in the butt. When she lived on the outskirts of West Phoenix, her home was over-sprayed (pesticides meant for crops accidentally applied elsewhere) by crop dusters and she swore her kids had developed chemical sensitivities (I suspect she was pretty normal even then, but probably not. She was an artist — my mother is an artist and definitely not normal). Sadly, she also had some trust that her government would assist her with protecting her family and others from experiencing future episodes of the same kind. I believe this is what made her a wild woman. Of course, Arizona's Pesticide Review Board could do little to help. Even if they could find evidence identifying a perpetrator, they had little ability to jerk someone's license for a single offense. Maybe a $100 fine. Strike one.

The Arizona Agricultural and Horticultural Commission (as the Arizona Department of Agriculture was then known) wouldn't create, let alone enforce, regulations that would force farmers to limit pesticide use. These agencies exist in every state. They are called the "State Lead Agency" (SLA) by their authorizing agency, the USEPA. They are authorized to enforce the Federal Insecticide, Fungicide, Rodenticide Act. The act originally was meant to protect the pesticide consumer from ineffective pesticides, but now basically requires manufacturers to test and register pesticides, and users to follow the label on the pesticide container (remember when I said it was the law?). It doesn't say anything about requiring a farmer to use alternate methods to prevent unnecessary, but legal, applications of a registered pesticide. More than once I have heard these agency officials state that it must be okay to use pesticides because the USEPA registers them. So Maude's neighbors had the right to use as much pesticide as they wanted, and the SLA wasn't going to do anything about it. Strike two.

Maude is not soft spoken. She got her story in the local papers and developed relationships with other mothers who believed their children were sick or in danger of becoming sick because of manmade toxins — air pollution, groundwater contamination, hazardous waste facilities and pesticides. They went to the Arizona Department of Environmental Quality (ADEQ) for help. "Stop killing our babies!" Environmental agencies, all authorized by the USEPA to help states implement federal environmental laws (Clean Air Act, Clean Water Act, etc.), have three basic functions: To issue environmental permits, monitor possible polluting entities (businesses and municipalities) for compliance with environmental regulations, and enforce compliance. In many states these agencies are under tremendous political pressure to permit pollution, keep the USEPA "off our backs", and "make sure business continues, comes and grows for the creation of jobs (votes) in our state." Maude and her pals forced ADEQ to pay attention to what it was supposed to do. But the agency couldn't stop polluters from coming to town and operating if those applying for permits had the money and lawyers to jump through all the hoops. "Sorry, Maude, we'll listen but can't do much..." Like most folks in government, whoever said things like this to Maude needed some lessons in risk communication. They had just created a "super-activist". Strike three!

And I was the ombudsman for ADEQ, the first state agency, environmental ombudsman in the U.S. An eccentric old U.S. Congressman named Sam Steiger thought up the idea – better communication between a state environmental agency and those it protects and regulates. Too bad more states haven't figured it out. The main function of an ombudsman is to communicate with people outside the agency who have a problem with the agency, then analyze and report that communication to decisionmakers in the agency. I was a "trouble shooter" appointed by the governor to work for the Director of ADEQ. I came to the agency about a year after Maude decided ADEQ was "full of bull..." (I love Maude. She sings my favorite song — John Mellencamp's "I fight authority and authority always wins".)

In 1991 I met Maude, and asked what all ombudsmen should ask, "What can I do to help you?" After she told me I was probably just another "industry toady", she said she had heard I was an entomologist for the University of Arizona and asked if I could help her stop her children's

13

new school (she had since moved to North Phoenix to get away from agriculture) from spraying insecticides in the classrooms.

Fat, dumb and happy as a "bug man for the U"

Months after finishing my graduate education in 1981 at The Auburn University, I was able to move back home to Tempe, Arizona, where I was to begin my job as an Integrated Pest Management (IPM) Specialist for the University of Arizona's Entomology Department. Having a Cooperative Extension (back then we called it the Agricultural Extension Service) appointment, I was based out of the Maricopa County Extension Office — actually just next door to where I worked four years prior as a "field grunt" for the US Department of Agriculture's (USDA), Animal, Plant Health Inspection Service (APHIS). The same folks who brought taxpayers eradication programs for Fire Ants, Screw Worm, Boll Weevil and the Mediterranean Fruit Fly. I worked on my hands and knees (literally) counting caterpillars on cotton and rangeland grasses so entomologists could figure out how to eradicate them. That experience taught me that if I wanted to make any meaningful decisions about pest management as an entomologist I would have to get a graduate degree.

In addition to containing the largest city in the state (Phoenix), Maricopa County had the largest agricultural production in the state. At that time Arizona was the third largest cotton producer in the U.S. Our irrigated farms produced some of the highest yields and best quality cotton in the world. Cotton was King! I was a Prince —or thought I was — and privileged for damn' sure. I was going to work with farmers and play with bugs. I loved the American Farmer and couldn't wait to become a helpful part of the system.

As a courtesy, Monday morning I reported to the County Extension Director. My real boss was the state IPM coordinator, Dr. Leon Moore in Tucson. The director welcomed me into his office and asked what program I would like to provide to his farmers. "Well sir, my job is to demonstrate and coordinate an IPM program in cotton. Leon tells me that the budworms are so resistant to methyl parathion they can damn' near swim in it before they eat." The "good ol' boy" County Extension Director looked at me (all six-foot-seven of him) and said as serious as a heart attack, "Marc, you go out there and tell those boys what insecticide to use, but don't start that IPM crap. IPM is communism."

I was a damn' scientist and I was damned if I was going to have some good ol' boy (actually the "good ol' boy" was a pretty fine plant pathologist in his day) tell me what was best for me — after all I knew what was best

— my professors at Auburn had taught me so. Sure. So, I said, "Yes, sir." And so I started out my nine years as an IPM Specialist working with our cotton agents and helping cotton growers figure out how to make the most of their insecticides.

I shared an office with Dr. Dave Langston. Dave's official Cooperative Extension responsibilities were livestock and urban pest management. He's a real people person, a farm boy from Oklahoma who loves telling stories and making folks laugh. Seems like half the day Dave would field phone calls from homeowners regarding the different pest problems they were having. Typical Phoenix urban pests: sewer roaches, scorpions, black widow spiders, Indian house crickets, house flies, mosquitoes, etc. Dave was good. He would tell folks what conditions were causing their pests, and what they should do to prevent them. This seemed to be more fun than killing bugs on cotton to me. In fact, my emphasis in entomology as a graduate student was in Medical Entomology: That's the study of human maladies caused by arthropods (bites, stings, diseases, and actual infestations such as maggots — yes, the sub-specialty forensic entomology "bugs on dead people" fall into "Med Ent" - neat stuff) and how one might manage those pests. I worked on the Red Imported Fire Ant for my graduate thesis. Urban pest management is closely related, but also includes stored product (flour beetles, meal moths, etc.) and structural (e.g., termites and carpenter ants) pests, as well as nuisance pests (e.g., ants, bees, flies, and silverfish). It was just fun dealing with pest problems that most of us live with daily.

I really enjoyed watching and listening to Dave work. In a lot of ways, it was then that I learned that "pest management is people management." Educating folks about their problems and convincing them that they can do something about them is a special skill. However, I also began to develop a real curiosity regarding just HOW one gets folks to adopt a new behavior. I remembered my dad (an old fashioned-pediatrician) telling me it takes not only medicine, but also the laying on of hands to heal folks, to make them believe that they can be healed. I had no real idea how to do this. Entomologists are not trained to change people, but to study bugs.

While Dave seemed to be making somewhat of a difference, I was getting nowhere convincing farmers to adopt ways other than massive pesticide applications, to control their pests. They weren't buying what I was selling — Integrated Pest Management.

Integrated Pest Management (IPM) DEFINED AS AN INNOVATION TO BE ADOPTED: IPM is a cluster of technologies (cultural, mechanical, biological, genetic, and chemical) which is an integrated application (based on biological information) designed to allow humans to compete with other species (pests).

In the practical sense, the concept of IPM goes to what environmental management professionals call pollution prevention. Born from concern about negative effects of hazardous waste on human health and the environment, environmental officials began discussing pollution in terms of waste. In short, there is "point source" pollution emitted from smokestacks and drainpipes, and other "non-point source" pollution from less defined or mobile sources. From this viewpoint, pesticides are a unique non-point source pollutant. They are intended to be applied to the environment, as opposed to other pollutants which are viewed as byproducts of civilization —or waste. Pesticide use that results in unnecessary costs, pollution or adverse health effects is inherently a management/people problem. IPM, in fact, is one of the oldest pollution prevention programs (though not historically termed such) for non-point source pollution. IPM is recognized by the USEPA and USDA as a viable cluster of technologies that prevent non-point source pollution and reduce pest management costs.

Even today, IPM has not fully diffused/been adopted by communities in the agricultural or urban sectors (GAO-01-815, 2001). I began to understand while trying to work with my farmers in Arizona that it was unlikely IPM would fully diffuse until it was, at least partially, diffused by the general population. And so I began to realize that implementing IPM in the public schools of the United States would initiate (and possibly accomplish) this diffusion. Unfortunately, many Land Grant/ Cooperative Extension institutions (the traditional implementers/change agents for IPM) either did not view the implementation of IPM in public schools as part of the extension mission, or were unwilling to jeopardize existing relationships regarding their Urban Pest Management programs of working with pesticide manufacturers and exterminators. Clearly, it was communication and the "laying on of hands" that was needed for the successful implementation of IPM, and this type of implementation seemed to me a lot more feasible in our schools than on our farms. When Maude finally got around to asking, I was ready.

16

PART II:
Solutions

Chapter Three – What our Children Deserve – "Just do the right thing."

The reason pests are managed in schools is to make the school environment a safe learning environment. The presence of pests in school buildings can represent both a threat to occupant health — through envenomization, allergic response or disease transmission — and a distraction from the learning environment. How many of us remember the disruptive effect of the lone, foraging paper wasp that happened to fly into our classroom on a warm spring afternoon, the mouse running across the floor or perhaps the cockroach on the wall or on the teacher's desk during a lecture? The specter of "sick school syndrome" that results in costly building closures, site remediation and negative public perception has sensitized administrators to the effects of toxic materials used, stored or propagated (as with molds) in their schools. Now more than ever, the routine use of pesticides in and around schools (landscape and turf) is, or should be, a concern of parents, teachers and school administrations (Goldman, 1995, Eskenazi, et. al., 1999).

Ask any pediatric toxicologist. Ask your Congressmen who crafted the Food Quality Protection Act (FQPA). Children are not just little adults! Yes, they are smaller, BUT their nervous systems are still developing — those things in our bodies that give us cognition and coordination. Most of the pesticides we use are NERVE POISONS and biocides (able to kill any organism if in large enough concentrations). For sure, many of the pesticides (organophosphates: e.g., diazinon, malathion, Orthene®) that you and I were brought up on are the direct descendents of World War I nerve gases and the Holocaust. Others (organochlorines: e.g., DDT and Chlordane) are poisons that Rachel Carson illustrated in *Silent Spring*, now proven to have killed, mutated or driven to extinction whole species of invertebrates and vertebrates. Guess what? Humans are vertebrates!

Some of those pesticides are still in use — in our schools. However, most of the pesticides used in our schools and homes today (synthetic pyrethroids, growth inhibitors, etc.) have active ingredients that seem to be less dangerous. However, the jury is still out on the effect of "endocrine disruptors" on humans. Perhaps of more immediate concern is how the inert ingredients, with which the active ingredients are mixed will affect us and our children (information which, by proprietary law, the manufacturers don't have to share with us). Oh, for you "organic" folks out there: What makes you think pesticides made from plants aren't poison? One of the oldest insecticides that we used in this country was Blackleaf 40 made from tobacco. It was banned years ago. As I mentioned before, pesticides have their place protecting us and allowing us to compete with pests. However, why would we use any of these toxins if we don't need to?

The school community (students, parents, teachers, administrators, elected officials, maintenance workers, custodial staff, kitchen staff, secretaries and nurses) demands a safe learning environment. They don't want pests in the school environment. On the other hand, a school community does not want to be exposed to toxins. That is a tough situation when you think about the traditional ways of controlling pests in schools — and the erroneous belief that pesticides prevent (not kill) pests. By integrating other strategies such as cultural control (sanitation) and mechanical control (exclusion) as the primary management strategies, and relegating chemical control to an as-needed strategy based on monitoring, schools can effectively address their demands of No Pests, No Toxins.

Minimum Standards for the Implementation of Integrated Pest Management in our Schools?

- The school administration is aware of what its pest management program is.
- Those responsible for cultural (sanitation) and mechanical (exclusion) components of IPM have been trained to incorporate them into existing job responsibilities.
- Those responsible for the chemical pesticide component of IPM are certified Pest Control Operators (with instructions to treat as needed and based on monitoring).

Is your school administration aware of what its pest management program is?

Call and ask! While the newest data from New York (Braband, Horn and Sahr, 2002) indicate that a majority of school districts have pest management policies and most require inspections, monitoring and record keeping, these are POLICIES resulting from either state mandates or the threat of state mandates (as in Indiana). In Indiana, Texas and Michigan, if you ask them they will say they have it covered, that they have a "pest management plan". But are they IMPLEMENTING a verifiable IPM program? NO!

Sure, school district administrators know how to respond to surveyors regarding the use of pesticides in their schools. But YOU call them and ask them. Ask them the specific questions I pose for "minimum standards for the implementation of pest management in schools" (see Appendix A), and let them know you are part of their school community and are WATCHING.

Over the last 10 years we have asked schools (through their district offices), "What are you doing to control pests in your schools?" More than 80% didn't have a clue. They could not tell us what pests they had, what was being done to control them (including what, if any, pesticides were being used), or whether the individual applying pesticides actually held a license to control pests. Notably, though, today many school systems are required to have Material Data Sheets (MSDS) on site when applying pesticides, some of the more progressive school districts are required to notify the school community about pesticide application and a few are required to have an IPM plan on record.

Have you ever read an MSDS? It is very technical, and either will confuse you or scare the hell out of you. I bet that if you call your school district it won't be able to find it in a timely manner and sure won't be able to explain it to you. The requirement to notify parents when pesticides are applied in schools is just for certain pesticides —many are exempt for toxicological (low mammalian toxicity presumed to be the AI in most insecticidal baits and gels) and emergency use (e.g., Killer Bees, Yellow Jackets, disease vectoring mosquitoes) reasons. The school board and school administrators' association lobbyists whined big time that this is an unfunded mandate. And it is! If they would spend their money preventing pests rather than spraying for them:

1) They wouldn't have to pay for the labor (applications) and materials (pesticides); and

2) They wouldn't have to buy postage and pay for administrative assistance to notify you that your children are being exposed to pesticides.

Remember what I said about management in Chapter One? If your management system demands pesticides, you will use them and you will pay for them. Pesticides really work. They kill pests — if the applicator knows where they are and when they might be most susceptible! But you don't have to kill pests when you can prevent pests. School districts I have worked with to utilize IPM have consistently been able to reduce their pesticide use by at least 90% and reduce pest complaints by at least 85% without increasing costs over a three-year period. Finally, we arrive at a depressing irony: the required IPM plan (e.g., in Michigan and Texas) each school district must have is a great idea, but unfortunately it's an unfunded mandate in most states. Walk in and ask to see the plan and have the district facilities manager, superintendent or your school's principal explain it to you. Most have it written for them by their contractor (i.e., the exterminator company) and have no idea what it is about — just another plan turned "manual" that your tax money paid for, now great at gathering dust.

Figure 1:
The traditional pest management model

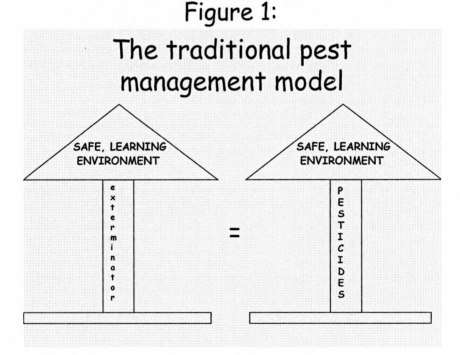

Are those responsible for the cultural (sanitation) and mechanical (exclusion) components of IPM trained to incorporate them into existing job responsibilities?

IPM does not have to cost more than traditional extermination programs. The IPM approach can be successful in the school environment because cultural (practices to reduce attracting pests) and mechanical (practices to exclude pests) strategies can be incorporated into existing custodial and maintenance activities. These include sanitation, energy conservation, building security and infrastructure maintenance. Monitoring efficiency (verification of pest presence) is enhanced via the virtual full-time presence and perception of the school's human inhabitants. This strategy relies on an educational approach that creates awareness in all occupants of a proactive management strategy, versus the reactive strategy of chemical treatment. Thus, by incorporating IPM into existing school operations (sanitation, maintenance and classroom education) and partnering with a qualified Pest Management Professional as a consultant/educator (rather than as an "exterminator"), school districts can overcome their natural resistance to "adding pest management to an already full plate".

"Do what you are doing now, just think pests"

The way I get these overworked and underpaid (I mean it!) members of the school community to even consider implementing IPM is to say, "Do what you're doing now, just think pests." What training program does your school district have that would allow custodians, maintenance workers, kitchen staff and teachers (all of whom have paid days for professional improvement programs) to become part of an IPM program? Such professional improvement programs have emerged for topics such as HIV and school security (post-Columbine).

Custodians clean, they straighten up the classrooms (yes, I remember my dad telling me to "straighten up your room!"), sanitize to prevent germs, repair or report broken windows, doors, etc. If they are provided with proper information they can easily:

- Recognize and reduce "harborage" (places where pests can eat, sleep and reproduce without being detected)
- Recognize and reduce unsanitary conditions (spilled or unsealed food and water that attract pests)

In short, they can "do what they are doing now" and prevent pests (including molds).

They are incorporating pest management into their jobs. It is the same for our friends in the kitchen. Is sanitary food prepared under sanitary conditions? Are they storing food in conditions to prevent germs? Does the food have bug and mice poop in it? Sanitation and clutter control — those things are already their job! They just need to know what they can do to prevent bugs and mice.

Maintenance workers provide structural integrity to the school environment so our children don't hurt themselves. In most school districts they maintain an energy management system that keeps cold air out in cold weather and hot air out in warm weather. These days they manage mold in the schools with controlled air flow and water damage control. Whatever they are doing for those activities relates to excluding pests from the school facility or preventing pests via reducing damp habitat. Weather-stripping, door brushes, caulking (actually, specific sealants dependent on the substrate), repaired windows, water leaks, etc. All exclude pests. If you can see daylight beneath an exterior door, roaches can enter the building. If you can fit a pencil under a door, a mouse can crawl through the same space. "Do what you are doing now, just think pests".

All members of the school community have the job of providing security for our children. Each has had some training to react to two-legged invaders: how to keep them out, detect them and what to do if they're spotted. I ask administrations to let these people learn about the four-, six-, eight and more-legged invaders they should keep out, detect and react to. Who better to observe these invaders than the inhabitants of the schools? If education is the foundation for IPM, monitoring is the backbone of IPM. What pests are present? Where are they and are they numerous enough to constitute a real problem?

School districts are essentially centralized and linear in their management hierarchy. While district administrators agree to implement IPM, that commitment must be demonstated by their willingness to communicate with principals, teachers, students, maintenance, custodial and kitchen staff. Whereas administrators and teachers normally are viewed as education professionals, the staff who are relied on to conduct cultural, mechanical and sometimes chemical control are not. Custodial staff are often long-term community members who take justifiable pride in their jobs. If communicated with as professionals and given control of pest management activities in their schools, they become more committed to the goals of the program.

It is interesting to note that custodians view teachers as responsible for attracting and harboring pests, and rightfully so. This viewpoint is not surprising when we consider that of all the individuals in the community, teachers are the only true, long-term human inhabitants of the school buildings. They with their possessions spend the most time in the facility. Teachers create an ideal habitat for pests via storing and consuming food products (for themselves, their students and classroom pets), propagating and maintaining house plants and developing (sometimes over decades) a "refugia" of collectables best categorized as clutter.

Of course, students are second only to teachers in their ability to provide transportation of pests to the school and provide sustainable harborage in the facility (e.g., lunch bags, lockers and even wheelchairs). It is my observation that teachers understandably behave in the school somewhat differently than in their homes, in that they rely on custodial staff to provide "house cleaning" functions. I mean, wouldn't you modify your behavior (become a bit less fastidious) if you had a custodian come to your home every day? This attitude could be viewed as the major barrier to effective pest-related communication in this centralized system. The good news is that because of the educational culture inherent in the school community, all community members can be receptive to informational communications that affect the consequences to one's actions—a common classroom phrase.

Figure 2:
current support system for public schools

SAFE, LEARNING ENVIRONMENT

custodial | maintenance | kitchen | Admin | students teachers

education

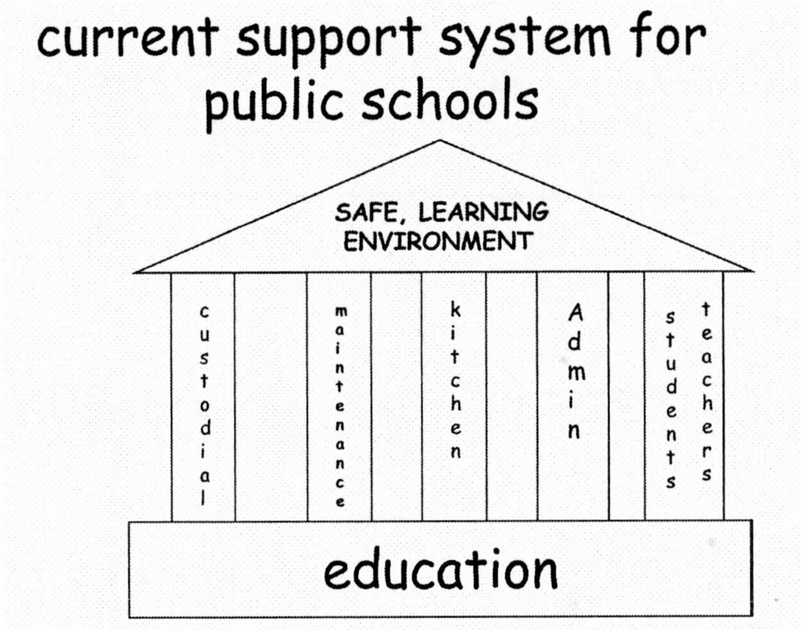

Are those who are responsible for the chemical pesticide component of IPM certified Pest Control Operators (with instructions to treat as needed and based on monitoring)?

As I have already mentioned, most schools in the country still have exterminators, on contract, "inspecting" once a month. While it is true that many of these Pest Control Operators are not specifically contracted to treat the school monthly, it is my observation that they do. Here is how it works: Your school district facilities manager takes the "low bid" for pest management from a local exterminator…say $350 per school per year. For this, the exterminator fully treats the school once annually (normally in the summer — treating the baseboards of all rooms and often the external perimeter cracks and crevices). Then every month during the school year the applicator spends about 45 minutes to one hour "inspecting" the school (which is really inadequate). They call that monitoring. Horse pucky. More often than not, they apply pesticides only where the teacher or head custodian tells them to.

In most of these low bid contracts the exterminator can get paid for "additional treatment". If you look at the invoices to the school district, every time these guys visit, they end up treating some alleged potential problem site. This practice can double the yearly contract cost, but it doesn't show up as a line item on the districts' contractual budget sheet! So, yeah, they will tell you they have inspected, monitored and treated on an as-needed basis, but who knows? Who is watching the store? We will get to that under "What is IPM…"

Are these guys really qualified to act as Pest Management Professionals? Almost never. IF they are certified (by passing a test given by the SLA on the safe use of pesticides) Pest Control Operators, does that mean they are trained and experienced in:

- Knowing the common pests for each particular school environment?
- Identifying each of those pests, as well as other less common pests?
- Identifying the conditions that attract or harbor (conducive conditions) each of those pests?
- Monitoring for the type of pest, specific areas in which they might be located and extent of the pest infestation in those areas? (see Appendix B)
- Applying all technical options (integrating pest management techniques) in each situation?

- Communicating all of the information above regarding pest problems and solutions to the appropriate school community member?

Unfortunately not (we will discuss the specifics of what a Pest Management Professional actually is, in the next chapter). Many Pest Control Operators just pass the test. It is my experience that some of these folks are trained and experienced in IPM, but they do only what they have time for (which is damn' hard under a low bid). Most states still allow Pest Control <u>Technicians</u> to "inspect" schools and apply pesticides. They work under the "supervision" of Pest Control Operators (who needn't be on-site). They might be trained to pretty much safely apply pesticides, are paid much less than Pest Control Operators and often have little experience or training required to be a real Pest Management Professional. Often, this is the "McJob" of the pest control industry. IT'S NOT THEIR FAULT. Your school district administration should know and approve what real IPM is and who practices it. Ask them if they do!

Figure 3:

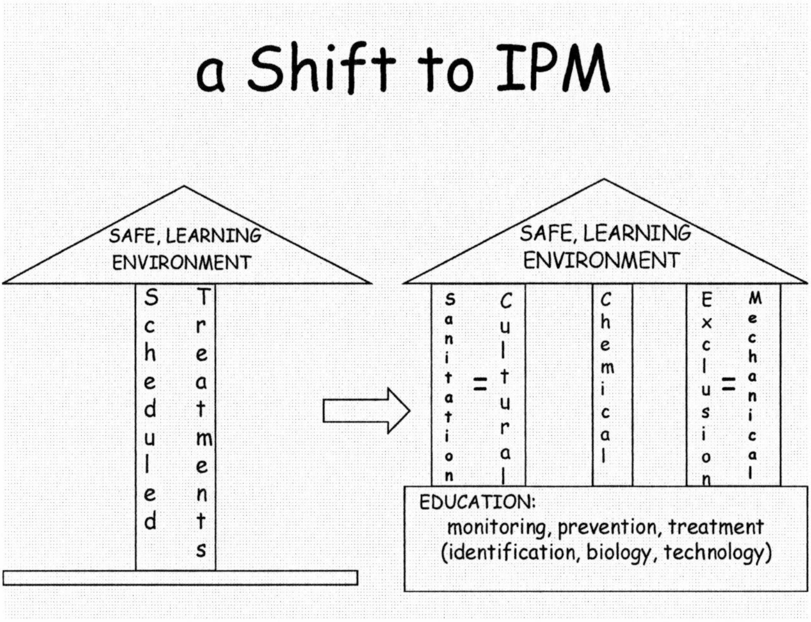

a Shift to IPM

Reality check for parents and school officials #1 - What IPM (figure 3) is:

- A management strategy based on communication/education supported by a committed school administration.

In fact, one of the major determinants for success when implementing IPM in schools is that the administration is doing this because "it is the right thing to do". But words are cheap. All major players in the school district feel like they already have too much on their plates. In this centralized system, leadership from the top is the key to commitment. These political animals (school board members and their district superintendents) know that policies without plans (strategies) are worthless,

Some of these folks will "glad hand" you all the way out the door while waving their IPM policy for review. Find out if they have communicated their IPM policy, with a logical and reasonable strategy for achieving its goals, to school principals, custodial supervisors, food service managers, kitchen managers and maintenance supervisors sufficiently that these site-based managers can incorporate IPM into the existing functions of faculty and staff. Have they committed to a training or educational program for school staff and/or faculty? If not, the program will not work or, at best, will be less than effective.

- A "partnership" of the school community (including concerned parents) with a qualified Pest Management Professional (figure 4).

I will write this again and again, but the only way this type of program will work is if the pest management contractor (a.k.a., the exterminator) is converted to a "Diagnostician/Educator". I have already described the minimum qualifications for the Pest Management Professional. If contractors are genuinely to conduct an IPM program for schools, they MUST be able to work with the people in those schools in order to deliver an effective program.

Custodians, kitchen staff, administrators, school nurses, (ideally, teachers and maybe students) need to be educated to allow the Pest Management Professional to diagnose the pest problem and conditions causing it (see Appendix C). These school inhabitants need to know what a Pest Vulnerable Area (PVA) is (e.g., kitchens, biology labs, TEACHER LOUNGES and custodial closets), and how to use and report the results of monitoring traps (Appendix B). They should be able to competently ask:

- Have you had any pest problems?

- What kind of pests are involved?
- Where are you noticing these pests?; and,
- For how long?

These questions (and more) are key to the diagnosis and require access to and education of the school community, just as your medical doctor can make a more accurate and timely diagnosis when you are available to answer questions and you are informed about your health issues. Conversely, what good is an MD who doesn't take the time (or managed care organization that doesn't allow your MD the time) to educate you and communicate with you? That person is unprofessional, unqualified or both!

Figure 4: A Shift to "Partnering" for Pest Management

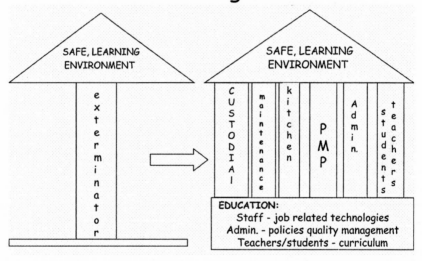

The Pest Management <u>Professional</u> must be able to identify a receptive audience in order to remediate conducive conditions. This professional can't help prevent or control pests in the school if the school community won't provide cultural control with better sanitation (less clutter in storage areas and classrooms, control over food in the classroom, fewer vending machines, improved cleaning techniques, etc.), and mechanical control with better exclusion (e.g., door sweeps, the proper sealant for foundation cracks and sealable food containers) any more than an MD can prevent or treat your disease if you are not taking care of yourself! These are management functions that the Pest Management <u>Professional</u> (or MD in the case of your health) can only recommend. It is up to the school officials to implement them. If the conditions that attract pests or allow access to pests are not managed, the chemical pesticides the professional might have to use will be of no more value than taking antibiotics for your respiratory infection will keep you from dying from cancer if you keep smoking.

- An educational system which empowers the school inhabitants to eliminate or reduce the reasons for insects, rodents and plants to become pests

As I have mentioned, the school inhabitants ultimately are responsible for creating an environment that does not attract pests... along with learning:

- How to identify a pest (is it a Praying Mantis or a roach?),
- How many of those pests might constitute an infestation (was it a single adult roach or many, or were there immature roaches?), and
- How to report their findings to the Pest Management <u>Professional</u>.

These school inhabitants (administration, staff, teachers and students) should have some education through in-service training and/or periodic newsletters which will empower them to know what conditions might attract pests to the school environment. These include improperly stored human or pet food, spilled food or drinks, improper waste management, filthy drains, pet feces, outside lights directly above external doors, water leaks, even warm temperatures.

- An educational system which empowers school inhabitants to prevent pests from entering the school facility

Once teachers, custodians, kitchen staff, nurses and administrators learn how to minimize the school's attractiveness to pests, they can also learn what parts of their job responsibilities can, in fact, keep the vermin out. Is it any wonder that Yellow Jackets (paper wasps) enter the school at the beginning of the school year when the soda pop syrup they love so much is in the open trash containers, placed directly outside the external doors that are left open to provide airflow at summer's end? What is attracting them and how are they getting in? It's all part of a cause and effect training program that occurs so often when schools encounter two-legged invaders.

- An educational system that empowers the school staff to know when to remedy and how to remedy documented pest problems by integrating cultural, mechanical and lowest-impact chemical control technologies

Teachers can accurately report pest problems, reduce harborage in the form of classroom clutter and use sealable containers for their in-class refreshments and teaching materials such as pet food, macaroni art, etc. They can teach students not to accidentally bring household pests to school. Custodians should be empowered to report data from monitoring traps and report conditions which would allow pests access to the school (poor weather-stripping, absent or broken screens and leaking pipes) just as they would report any other maintenance problem. They should clean from the pest point of view rather than from the less-observant human view. Maintenance workers replace or repair doors, windows and pipes as part of their building safety and energy management functions. Kitchen staff should use sealable containers for food, boxless storage to reduce clutter and cardboard (roaches love cardboard – it provides both shelter and food), replace dark shelving and pallets with wire shelving and order supplies only from uncontaminated vendors. Administrators write (or sign) work orders for better equipment and maintenance response. They can write and enforce policies to reduce classroom clutter, cease doing business with sloppy and/or contaminated vendors (improper trash storage containers and pick-up, leaking vending machines, infested food supplies), replace dangerous chemicals with lower-impact baits and inform parents about these actions. It's all part of a well-managed school that already must satisfy OSHA, local health inspectors, parents and the school board... but now by JUST THINKING PESTS!

Reality check for parents and school officials #2 - What IPM is NOT:

- A term or job description added to that of an unwilling or unqualified individual (the school district must either employ or contract with a qualified Pest Management Professional).

Who is your school district's IPM coordinator? As I have mentioned, some of your school districts have them. Just what qualifies them to "coordinate" your pest management program? Are they people who were picked because the school superintendent needed to name someone according to the new policy, or did they volunteer? Why did they volunteer? Are they believers in IPM or just looking for a boost in pay? What is their training related to pest management and are they licensed? Do they really know what IPM is and how to practice it?

Nearly all pest control "specialists" I meet, whether contracted or in-house, tell me they are practicing IPM. Many are not licensed, and even if they are, too many of these guys couldn't tell you the difference between a Pharaoh Ant and a Pavement Ant, a Deer Mouse and a House Mouse, an organophosphate and pyrethroid insecticide. And they damn' sure couldn't begin to discuss the proper monitoring trap placement for German Cockroaches in school kitchens. Perhaps the most common and pervasive misinformation these guys lay out is that they are implementing an IPM program when, in fact, all they have done is switched from spraying baseboards to applying cockroach or ant baits. While I appreciate the change to lower impact, probably more effective insecticides, this is substitution - NOT integration. What horse pucky! Later you will read some real horror stories about what schools and their employees or contractors are doing in the name of IPM.

- A "low bid" process subject to unqualified exterminators, or qualified Pest Management Professionals who will not be able to perform to professional standards

I cannot say enough bad things about the requirement of schools, where our children reside for six hours a day (sometimes eight hours if they are part of extended day programs), that have to accept the lowest bid to manage sometimes dangerous pests with sometimes dangerous pesticides. I have mentioned that, at the very least, this forces the Pest Management Professional to under-bid in order to win a contract. They become professionals who know how to diagnose and educate, but cannot afford the time to do anything but revert to the 1960s pest management practices of scheduled spray applications. Of course, one could argue that these professionals should not take on jobs that will not allow them to practice up to their profession's standards.

The most common result of the low bid is that pest control companies normally will send underpaid and under-trained "technicians" to apply pesticides. It's perfectly legal. If it weren't so much fun to listen to these guys answer pest management questions, I would recommend that this practice be outlawed in facilities that house children. In fact, yes, let's outlaw this practice! However, don't blame it all on them. These guys are told to spray and that's what they do. In fact, school staff will force them to spray. They even are told to spray kindergarten room carpet for lice! I know decisionmaking individuals in schools who won't pay exterminators if they "can't smell the poison" after their visit.

32

The most egregious results of the low bid are unlicensed contractors or school employees (no bid) who have been told to "get some bug juice and spray the school" by managers who just don't care. These individuals have been known to spray extremely toxic, agricultural –use-only, pesticides in classrooms because they didn't want to spend money on registered products or because that's what they did "down home" —spray into air ducts during school hours or pour gasoline into a nest of Yellow Jackets next to a school building. This negligence is a result of horrible management by the school administration.

The low bid does not have to be. School districts can afford to have Pest Management Professionals conduct real programs IF they require or allow them to partner with trained school employees for pest monitoring and pest-conducive condition inspection. Thus, the Pest Management Professional would not have to spend more time at the school facility and the time he/she *does* spend would be as a diagnostician/educator or very occasionally, a low impact pesticide applicator. Under these conditions, school districts can require a Request for Qualifications (RFQ) which would act as a filter for Requests for Proposals. School districts also could audit their current pest management programs to develop actual costs (remember the difference between contract costs and call-back application costs) and compare these to those of a quality program, then budget for an efficient, cost- effective IPM program. The Bloomington, Indiana school system reduced its pests and pesticides by 90% while reducing costs by 35%.

- An "out of sight, out of mind" contractual function. The school community must be willing to communicate with its Pest Management Professional in order to facilitate long-term cultural controls (practices to reduce attracting pests) and mechanical controls (practices to exclude pests)

This point, of course, is related to the school district's and Pest Management Professional's willingness to partner on IPM. All the school districts that practiced traditional pest management relegated pest management to the "exterminator". The only time the administrator with control over that contract heard about it was either when the contract was up for renewal, when a school was being overrun by pests (at one school mice were literally dropping out of the ceiling onto students), or when the school had to be evacuated due to improper pesticide use. School districts and the Pest Management Professional should develop a Memorandum of Understanding to address this partnership (see figure 4). Further, those school business officials need to understand the importance of this type of service procurement. After all is said and done, IPM is a process, not a miracle, and all actors must be a part of that process or it just won't work.

- A chemical pesticide program to prevent pests from entering schools

Let's get this straight: In school buildings there is no such thing as a preventative chemical treatment for pests! It doesn't work, it is wasteful, it is harmful and it is a lie. In Las Vegas I had a national pest control company try to tell me it was practicing IPM by applying insecticide baits in and around the school kitchens annually. This was a required application with no regard to the necessary use of the chemical pesticide tool indicated by the presence or absence of pests. By now you know that this is what most schools and parents believe is needed and works — "spray and they won't come". Sometimes this works with our turf grass pests (particularly when we want our yards and football fields to resemble indoor green carpet), but for structural pest management, the preventive application of chemical pesticides is normally misuse of expensive and possibly dangerous toxins.

In structures, when used correctly, pesticides will kill pests in a given area as long as the pesticide is effective. Yes, there is a phenomenon called translocation among social insects (e.g., ants, bees, and termites) where the pesticide is carried back to the "colony", but the insecticide is controlling only an existing infestation, NOT preventing future infestations. Further, unlike the very persistent chlorinated hydrocarbons (DDT, Chlordane, et al.), current insecticides are not very persistent. Depending on the environment (temperature, UV light, humidity) these toxic agents provide lethal effects anywhere from minutes to weeks…sometimes months in the case of very well placed insecticide baits. Unfortunately, these baits have begun to fail due to increased resistance exhibited in some of our most common pest species. This, of course, is no surprise. As most scientists know, continuous exposure of adversity (toxins in this case) to organisms with a high generational turnover breeds resistance.

When living in Phoenix, I always was (and still am) amused by customers (homeowners and school officials) who pay exterminators to spray the outside perimeter of homes and schools before total darkness. Think! Daytime temperatures are 110 degrees during the day, with unshaded ground temperature somewhere around 180 degrees, and the ground stays real hot into the night. This temperature deactivates most chemicals within minutes of their use. Yeah, the pesticides will kill most pests they come in contact with, but in these very hot months most pests are not exposing themselves to these killer temperatures! **Timing and coverage are the keys to effective pesticide use**. If the pesticide is not used when it is most effective on what it is supposed to kill, it is a waste. It presents unnecessary exposure to humans and pets and it promotes a false sense of security with regard to dangerous pests.

- A no-chemical pesticide option. Situations do exist in which chemical pesticides are necessary and can be used safely.

Okay, now it is my turn to upset those who believe we can compete with pests for food, shelter, attention and public health, while living the suburban dream, without pesticides. E.O. Wilson (*Conservation Biology*, 1987) very eloquently explains that humans wouldn't be here without insects. They pollinate our food and sources of oxygen production, they decompose plants and animals to provide nourishing soil (not to mention acting as nature's garbage men), they provide medicine, clothes, shelter and (for most of the world's population) a significant part of their diet. Most people consciously eat bugs! If you ask me, bugs aren't competing with us. They are just taking what is already theirs! But, I AM AN ENTOMOLOGIST. I was that kind of kid and won't grow up.

Listen, folks; I love bugs. I can live with bugs. I don't mind eating them, sharing my food with them, even giving them some of my bodily fluids. I am okay knowing that most humans have mites (follicle mites) living on them – all the time! I am okay knowing that most of us will, at one time or other, have lice. My attitude is that when you have ecto-parasites you are never alone (more bug humor), and I am serious when I say I would much rather become food for baby flies and beetles (maggots and grubs) than be pumped full of formaldehyde when I die. I can sleep with them and go to the bathroom with them – BUT CAN YOU? Be honest. How many of you are that much into nature?

We all have different tolerance thresholds for pests. For some in my house the threshold for roaches and mice is zero, one or two for flies, three or four for ants. What is yours? Most of these thresholds have been established by the chemical companies so we use more chemicals — even deodorants for body odor tolerances. We of the Western World like to smell nice and not have bugs on us or around us. Read May Berenbaum's book, *Bugs in the System*. She does a great job of explaining this stuff. However, the bottom line is while there are some of us who can live with most pests, we won't allow ourselves to be killed by their bites, stings and diseases they transmit. Thus, sometimes chemical pesticides become part of the IPM strategy. While the vast majority of pest problems lend themselves to preventive strategies, ongoing and explosive pest infestations sometimes dictate the inclusion of chemical or biological pesticides in the IPM program. Your schools cannot tolerate massive roach infestations due to health codes, or because they might be asthmatic triggers, nor can they tolerate nests of "Africanized Bees" on or near school ground. There are a lot of examples of when pesticides should be used for safety or public health reasons and to "knock down" huge pest populations that the lack of preventive strategies allowed to flourish. Once they are controlled, a full IPM program (particularly the education as to why these infestations occurred) can be implemented. But make no mistake, if we and our children are to maintain the quality of life we have come to demand, chemical pesticides will remain part of modern pest management. But also make no larger mistake: Chemical pesticides should be used only as the last or only resort, based on necessity, with the lowest toxicity possible, applied assuring the least possible exposure, by a licensed, experienced pest manager and YOU HAVE A RIGHT TO KNOW ABOUT IT!

Memorandum of Understanding

Pest management challenges vary greatly among schools. There is also considerable variability among schools as to their levels of IPM expertise. Some schools have their own IPM coordinators. Others depend on Pest Management Professionals (PMPs) to catalyze the institutionalization of IPM. Most schools fall somewhere in between. This is why it is critical to the success of any school IPM program to begin with clear expectations, open communication and a dedication to promoting IPM education among all parties involved.

A Memorandum of Understanding (MOU) is a pre-contract document that defines the school/PMP relationship. Because IPM may have different meanings for different people, the MOU is a good way to make sure that both parties agree upon the goals and treatment strategies of the IPM program, in addition to understanding and communicating the correct expectations for the partnership they are about to form.

PMPs who practice true IPM are educated not only in the health, safety, handling, and application techniques related to pesticides, but also in the sanitation, biologic, genetic and mechanical aspects of pest control. The contractor must work as an educator, effectively communicating the steps that the school community should take on a regular basis to best manage pest problems. As such, many PMPs perform functions more akin to those of consultants than simply pesticide applicators.

Schools must commit to carrying out the recommendations of their IPM consultants. Through the MOU,

PMPs are credited for their knowledge of IPM and are empowered to make strategic pest management decisions. In the MOU, schools agree to abide by those decisions, in effect formally agreeing to hold up their end of the bargain. The MOU reinforces the commitment, education and communication components of IPM, which form the basis of the partnership.

Because schools want PMPs to provide a more comprehensive type of service, school administrators need to evaluate PMPs competing for contracts based more on their experience and expertise with IPM, than on how little the service will cost. That is not to say that cost should not be a factor. Rather, it should be one among many. With the paradigm shift from regularly scheduled monthly pesticide sprayings to the more proactive, comprehensive systems approach of IPM, there needs to be a corresponding shift in the manner in which PMPs are selected and contracted by schools.

Because successful IPM does not necessarily require regular monthly pesticide applications, the PMP may not need to visit on such a basis, once the program has been established. Visits may become quarterly, with school custodial, instructional, maintenance and kitchen staff taking the steps necessary to successfully maintain the IPM program. As time goes on and school staff become more accustomed to thinking about pests while performing their normal duties, the PMP may simply serve as an inspector or monitor who consults with school staff, occasionally applying pesticides in emergency situations. Compensation agreements should be structured accordingly.

Schools cannot simply hire a contractor and expect the firm to do away with all their pest problems. Successful IPM programs depend on school employees being conscious of pests as they perform their normal work responsibilities. Keeping areas clear of clutter and fixing leaky pipes are good examples. At the same time, it is the responsibility of the PMP to thoroughly inspect the school premises and suggest solutions to pest problems, such as moving dumpsters a minimum distance away from school doors. Both sides must commit to holding up their end of the partnership.

The MOU goes beyond the monetary commitment to IPM; it goes to the management commitment. IPM is a management issue, in terms of the behavior of the school community, the dedication of the PMP and the willingness of all involved to create a safer and healthier learning environment. An MOU helps to recognize the professionalism of the pest management industry and empowers the local PMP to make decisions that will be carried out.

In an attempt to be a sustainable management program, IPM seeks to internalize in the school as many pest management responsibilities and actions as possible. Schools can take simple steps to decrease their vulnerability to pests. Many times, this means changing old habits. The MOU works to achieve this, while relying heavily on the expertise of the PMP. Additionally, the commitment of both parties to the MOU will allow for cost-effective pest management.

Chapter Four – The Good, the Bad, and the Ugly

I have discussed the problems regarding pest management in our schools, how our society evolved to the state of chemical dependence we now find ourselves in and what the school community deserves — a committed, verifiable and cost-effective pest management program. If you have read closely, you will have noticed that I have not mentioned any serious technical or pest problems associated with IPM because technically managing pests in schools is usually no big deal. Experienced Pest Management Professionals can handle just about any pest, assuming they have the ability to use the tools that IPM provides. What I will spend most of this text explaining (and offering solutions for) are the problems with getting people to implement IPM. Again, "Pest management is people management".

I have alluded to or downright accused several groups of blocking IPM implementation in the school community and elsewhere. Indeed, I have spent little time discussing the heroes who risk their careers by pushing IPM, and I have been purposely fuzzy about those who just don't have their ducks in a row sufficiently to do what taxpayers are paying them to do. In this chapter I will discuss three basic groups of folks who should be implementing IPM. I categorize them as the Good, the Bad and the Ugly. As with any other groups of humans, it is difficult to categorize them as 100% good, bad, or ugly. However, I will try to put things into perspective for current users of pest management information and services, whether they are customers of the private or public sector.

The Good

In short, these people are risk takers. They are willing to ask strangers, or worse, friends and colleagues, to try something new. Sometimes they believe it to be their job, but often they just believe it to be "the right thing". They stand the risk of being rejected, ridiculed and perceived as a failure. As with many change agents who are willing to take risks, they are evangelical in their beliefs. They truly believe that implementing IPM will reduce risks to the school community of both pests and unnecessary pesticides. The "Good" folks I will discuss here are of the Demand Side or Supply Side persuasion. Sometimes they are both. They might be individuals who are offended by bad management, or greedy people. Mostly they are just very concerned and dedicated folks who want to do "the right thing".

- School Community Activists

Sometimes it's a concerned parent like Maude who just won't take no for an answer when it comes to her children, or a teacher who sees things that just aren't right or perhaps has developed a chemical sensitivity from years spent in the classroom. Maybe it is a group of high school students like those at Cass Technical High School in Detroit who took a science project and changed the way their school managed pests. Most of these activists are fairly low-key versus the in-your-face tactics of many others, although it takes all kinds.

John Carter of the Monroe County Community School Corporation (MCCSC) in Bloomington, Indiana, started out helping some of my graduate students assess the pest management practices of his school district. As a school business official, he had heard of IPM in 1994 but really didn't associate it with his job. However, he did occasionally hear about students and teachers who came down sick within days after their school was treated for pests. He did associate these absences with pesticides, but was unsure what he could do about it. When we presented him with a proposal to try IPM in his schools he jumped on the wagon and never wavered. Not only is MCCSC now regarded as a premier model of IPM (the "Monroe IPM Model"), but John assists school districts throughout the nation with implementation of that model, as well. He became our activist.

What is so great about school community activists is that they are peers of others in the school district in terms of being customers and professionals. These folks are mostly self- taught. They regard IPM as a management technique and are observant enough to know that traditional pest control is not good enough for them or their children. They recognize it is just bad management. Sure, guys like me can impress the hell out of members of the school community with our entomological terms and good looks, but peers are the people whom others in the schools relate to. These activists can relate the attributes of IPM to their peers in their own language and values.

I learned the hard way that, while health professionals or scientists can be convincing, nothing is more compelling to political decisionmakers than the image of a mother holding her child and begging for (or demanding) a safer environment for that baby. Arming this individual with the cost-effective facts of the IPM solution while they are pointing out the problem is an especially powerful strategy for dealing with decisionmakers. Those people are bombarded with problems, but seldom receive meaningful suggestions for solutions. You can imagine how well this works when it is carried out in conjunction with newspaper or TV coverage—and concerned parents are usually newsworthy! The old saying, "when you have them by the balls, their hearts and minds will follow", can and does work for driving policy. That's demand-side IPM.

- Organizations that Promote IPM

Several non-profit organizations with whom I have dealt are working hard and taking risks to move IPM higher on the local, state and national agenda. Some are professional coalitions dedicated to the broad application of IPM such as the National Foundations for IPM Education and the IPM Institute of North America, Inc. Some are local or national associations like Beyond Pesticides (formally known as the National Coalition Against the Misuse of Pesticides – NCAMP), Children's Health Environmental Coalition, Improving Kids Environment and a number of others who have organized and developed political clout they can use to demand better pest management in our schools.

I believe people like Mike Wallace, with the National Foundation for IPM Education, and Tom Green with the IPM Institute of North America, who have spent many years in agricultural IPM, are guys who just can't believe schools don't practice IPM. Mike is using his commodity group members to further this cause and is instrumental in moving IPM with his assistance in grants administration and political pandering. He has developed some great certification programs that identify just what real IPM is — whether in crops or schools. Without Tom's assistance, the EPA, many Pest Management Professionals and university urban entomologists wouldn't understand what verifiable means in terms of IPM. It is just too

41

easy for users to say, "Sure, we practice IPM." Yeah, prove it! Tom's IPM Star® provides the proof and rewards it.

Activists like Jay Feldman of Beyond Pesticides hold a special place in my heart. Jay has been there to kick my posterior a few times for not including groups like his in my initial attempts to bring school IPM implementers together. He helped teach me that I must reach beyond traditional implementers of IPM (Cooperative Extension, etc.) to develop strategies for national implementation. Beyond Pesticide newsletters provide some of the most comprehensive information about what is really happening with pesticides in our society. The Children's Health Environmental Coalition has been innovative by having celebrities like Olivia Newton John and Kelly Preston elevate awareness of children's environmental health. Awareness of that sort is absolutely critical to getting schools to adopt IPM.

The fact is, IPM will not diffuse into our culture without these dedicated activists. They are not scientists or regulators, but parents who care about children. My friend Tom Neltner, who as a former chemical engineer for a manufacturer and environmental attorney (and, like me, once an official in a state environmental agency), has become a ferocious advocate of children's health issues in the Midwest. In particular, Tom is largely responsible for developing and pushing through an IPM policy that almost all schools in Indiana now use; he's a meticulous and dangerous fighter. To my personal sense of amusement, Tom is not foolish enough to think that policies alone will implement IPM in schools. He actually has investigated schools in Indiana that are just "talking the IPM talk" and then delighted in bursting their fallacious bubbles. It is always a joy to watch these less-than-truthful school officials run for cover when confronted with their own deceptions. I had cautiously viewed the National Pest Management Association as willing to step up and take risks for our kids. I will discuss its mission and confusion next.

- Pest Management Professionals

Now that you know the difference between Pest Management Professionals and Exterminators, think about the risks these folks take when they tell their customers or potential customers, "If all you want is someone to spray pesticides in your school once a month, get someone else". By far, the majority of Pest Management Professionals are small businessmen. It is extremely difficult for them to turn down customers, but some do it. They believe in what they are supplying. Do you have any idea how easy it is for exterminators to "squirt and run", and how much money they can make – IF they don't bother to act as diagnosticians and educators? So, yes, they risk their competitive advantage by not taking the fast and easy way, and they also risk the scorn of traditionalists in their profession. Many traditionalists take pride in their belief that they have protected their customers from pests for many years. I believe that many of them have practiced pest control to the best of their ability, BUT within the framework of "one bug, one pesticide application" that entomologists from the universities and pesticide manufacturers have given them. Change is hard, and change can be dangerous to agents of change.

The best guys I know, like Dr. Bobby Corrigan and Larry Pinto, not only have excellent backgrounds in pest management, but also have training in facility sanitation and are fantastic educators. While these guys are rare commodities, many excellent Pest Management Professionals know what IPM is and how to apply it. Further, they often will take on projects that demonstrate their professionalism in worthwhile situations, without the motivation of profit. They know what "investment" means in terms of experience, goodwill and publicity, and eventually they will reap the benefits of their investment.

Of course, the vast majority of Pest Management Professionals out there are not going to hand you their Ph.D. diploma. Most of these professionals have spent thousands of hours as exterminators and/or training in academic fields related to pest management (entomology, plant science, zoology, etc). Some have no degrees and some have little experience. The good Pest Management Professional is a believer in IPM, enjoys applying the real thing and LOVES talking about it. Take Mike Lindsey in Arizona, who has lots of experience and worked in one of the original pilot cotton IPM programs back in 1968. Mike moves anyone he works with and is a super entomologist. He is "the man" when I want someone on the ground convincing classroom teachers to clean up their act. I saw him (when asked to testify about IPM in the early 90s) back down members of his state legislature with a "hissing roach" crawling on his shoulder and telling them in the parlance of the OK Corral (Tombstone, Arizona, is Mike's ancestral home) that he had been "waiting 15 years to meet you sum' bitches and now I got you".

By my definition, very few PMPs are employed by school districts. Jerry Jochim spent 11 years as maintenance and custodial staff for the Monroe County Community School Corporation. He earned his bachelor's degree at age 50 and was looking for some new work experience. After our initial pilot program at this Bloomington, Indiana, school district, we convinced (suckered) Jerry into becoming the IPM Coordinator for the 20 schools in the district. Jerry thought he didn't know squat about pest management, and indeed, he was vacant on bug knowledge, but he knew energy management, sanitation and the school community. Today he is a licensed Pest Control Operator and at least as good as the average PCO in the areas of bugs and pesticides. But he leaves them in the dust when it comes to understanding why pests are in schools and how to keep them out. He understands the dynamics of school structures as well as manageable square foot assignments for each custodian. In fact, he is often consulted by the best guys I know about these issues. He is a true believer, knows the real thing and LOVES talking about it. While he is still protecting our schools in Bloomington, his educational programs for custodians are being used all over the country.

In general, the national and large local pest control companies don't want to offer a real IPM program to school districts at an affordable price. Their business profit margin is based on volume. Occasionally, though, one of their PCOs decides or gets permission to control pests in schools at cost, as a community service. What is really neat about some of these guys is that once the profit motive is out of the equation, their latent desire to practice Professional Pest Management emerges. They take the time to figure out the right thing for the school and use their skills and experience to manage pests. I know a few who went wild and started self-teaching IPM.

Richard Lumpkin in Auburn, Alabama, worked for a large local pest control firm that provided fairly low-cost service to the school district. His boss told him to cooperate with us when we initiated the Monroe County IPM Model in Auburn. At first, Richard felt threatened by our program, but he was convinced to hang in there by Dr. Fudd Graham of the Auburn University Department of Entomology and Plant Pathology. Richard's pest management went from spraying the outside of buildings with gallons of pesticides monthly to using minimal amounts of roach bait when the traps indicated treatable infestations. Is he completely IPM? No, but damn' close and he is moving faster than we can keep up toward total implementation. He eats up all the IPM information we send him and wants all of his colleagues to convert. He owns his own business now and still protects the Auburn City Schools —still, I bet, offering his community service discount. I hear that his investment is paying off. Many of the teachers in the school district are asking him to manage pests at their homes — at full price. Richard is truly a poster boy for Pest Management Professionals when it comes to IPM in schools.

Scott, who works for a national chain that professes to protect your home's perimeter from killer bugs, also has been providing this community service to daycare centers in Bloomington, Indiana. Like Richard, he is an example of real professionalism. The guy would make a great entomologist.

He is fascinated by bugs and loves to talk about them. I hear he keeps Brown Recluse spiders in his home. Cool. We convinced him to change his daycare route from late evenings to daytime so he could communicate with daycare administrators and teachers. What a difference! — much better trap monitoring and fewer pest problems. Again, is he all the way there for IPM? No, but mostly so because he does not have the time, training or permission of his employers to convert to the real thing. I am sure that given the right circumstances he could be the industry poster boy for IPM in daycare facilities.

The bottom line is that nationwide implementation of IPM in schools and especially in daycare facilities cannot happen without Pest Management Professionals. It is my observation that school districts with more than 15 schools should seriously consider internalizing the PMP. Somewhere around 15 schools is the point at which school districts can afford to combine all IPM functions with other school operations. Imagine the efficiency of having the PMP as part of the school district's mid-level management team, with a continuous relationship with those who provide the cultural, mechanical and monitoring functions of the IPM program. Obviously, this arrangement is much more efficient, particularly in terms of education/training.

However, thousands of school districts throughout the U.S. are not large enough, lack money or are not managed well enough to internalize IPM functions. They use either untrained school employees or traditional exterminators to react to their pest problems. I have observed that many exterminators want to be real PMPs and practice real IPM if they feel it will not be a risk to their businesses. The best of these already have figured out that if they partner with school district personnel, they can decrease their time spent on monitoring, pesticide application and paperwork by allowing those in the schools to benefit from their diagnosis and education. They know they can charge the same for less, but more effective use of their time in each school district and use that saved time to increase their customer base. To this point, the National Pest Management Association (NPMA) represents many private pest control operators and almost all the national pest control companies in the U.S. In recent years, the administrative staff of the NPMA has tried really hard to develop professional standards for PCOs who deal with children's facilities. Indeed, they did partner up with Beyond Pesticides to sponsor legislation that mandates IPM in schools. In this they are attempting to increase the supply of school IPM-trained PCOs. Their education programs are quite good — and no wonder, seeing that Bobby Corrigan coordinated them. They are using the right words; unfortunately their actions contradict them.

When I began writing this book I wondered if the more powerful members of that association would ever really embrace this professionalism without trying to make the schools (taxpayers) shell out more than needed. In April of 2002 a group of school IPM implementers met with management of the NPMA to develop criteria and certification that would professionalize their members for school IPM. We were assured that a rigorous written exam and workplace standards would be developed for certification. Further, we were told that in-house professional pest managers employed by school districts would have access to such training and certification. Many of us worked to assist in developing these tools.

To date, those assurances have not materialized. The test questions developed by two of the most respected members of this association have either not been incorporated or are now part of a "self-testing" program. Professional standards have been relegated to labels and dress code (Quality Pro®) rather than incorporating nationally recognized standards for school IPM practitioners stipulated by Tom Green from the IPM Institute of North America. There has been no attempt to include non-pest control industry school employees who are real Pest Management Professionals in the ranks of this organization. As one of the world's leaders in urban IPM puts it, "The heart has been taken out of this program" (Anonymous, 2004). No doubt it is always about the money.

- "Heroes" and "Believers" in Government

What can I say? These are the folks who really could be moving this program. Unfortunately, as with many of our national issues, government is so large now that it hardly budges unless it is a political crisis. I will piss on their shoes in the "Ugly" part of this chapter, but suffice to say that many people in most government agencies are turf-bound and risk-averse. Fortunately, there are "believers" in government who have not only implemented the laws of this country, but also have read them enough to understand the intent of those laws. Some, like Al Greene with the Government Service Administration, are outstanding entomologists implementing cutting edge IPM in more buildings than I will ever crawl around in. Al is a true guru of structural pest management. Some of these folks, particularly in environmental agencies, understand how and why the USEPA was founded. They understand what the National Environmental Policy Act and subsequent environmental acts intended, and specifically the intent of the changes to FIFRA, post-Rachael Carson. Many are aware of the ironic lack of progress with the use of pesticides since *Silent Spring* stimulated so much other environmental progress. They know that there is a better way to manage pests and that it is the "right thing to do".

Rosemary O'Leary wrote an excellent article about the ability of mid- and lower-level government workers to overcome, or in some cases subvert, the environmental policies or lack of policies which adversely affect the public (O'Leary, 1994). In worst cases, some are whistleblowers, but in most instances "believers" quietly, legally and ethically overcoming the barriers erected by political appointees and anti-environmental lobbyists. I know government employees in local, state and USEPA Regional offices, as well as EPA headquarters in D.C. who, without agency policy or budgets, have been able to facilitate the progress we have made thus far. They used discretionary or generally directed funds under the authority of FIFRA. For obvious reasons I leave most of their names out of print, but these are people like Carl Martin in Arizona, brave beyond belief in standing up to a state agency that was all but captive to the pest control industry. Charles Moses with the state of Nevada went to the local newspapers to embarrass the Las Vegas schools into trying IPM. Larry Swain with the state of Michigan developed the famous program at Cass Tech High School and has applied it to the neediest intercity areas in his state. Retired USEPA, OPP "charter members" Bill Curry, Ralph Wright and Jim Boland (who called me his favorite foil because my mouth was "protected") have worked behind the scenes for years at some risk to move IPM into schools. They have, at an average cost of less than three SUVs per state (Kubista and Lame, 2003), been able to develop IPM in school informational materials (manuals, websites, brochures, etc) training programs and demonstration models that affect millions of children. They have sometimes done this by partnering with agency critics (offending administration supporters in the process) and working on their days off. They take risks and they fulfill their agency's mission to protect human health and the environment. I honor them.

- "Black sheep" of the Land Grant Universities

When I was a baby entomologist with the University of Arizona's Cooperative Extension Service I heard a motivational speaker at my first annual Extension conference in Tucson. He asked, "What kinds of people are Extension Agents (or Specialists)?" I think the guy was a sociologist. Anyway, he said research indicated that Extension folks are more akin to missionaries than any other profession. At the time I was slightly offended, as I never had much use for folks coming to my door on Saturday morning and trying to convert me to something I didn't want to understand (they were brave people, as I usually answered the door in my underwear, offering them a beer — not being mean, just ornery). However, after 10 years as an Extension Specialist and another 10 or so as an ex-patriot, I couldn't agree more with his premise. In fact, what I did as an Agricultural Extension Specialist was go out to farms in Arizona and try to convert farmers and their pest control advisors to the IPM religion. While I have never given up on that evangelical pursuit, I must admit that there were times I just told them what pesticides to apply and conducted my "field trials" for pesticide manufacturers (Dow, Pennwalt, Abbott, FMC, Shell, Union Carbide, American Cyanimid, and others) so Pest Control Advisers would have better products to kill pests with. As I related at the beginning of this book, that was what the County Agents wanted, the agricultural industry wanted and the Land Grant System (under the authority of the USDA) wanted...but what I truly wanted was to practice entomology in the fashion of the pest management teachings I learned in graduate school.

The system hasn't changed that much since I left in 1990. Extension Specialists still have to make their clients (County Agents, farmers, agribusiness, etc.) happy and generate grant monies by conducting field trials and publishing papers about the results of those trials. Urban pest management specialists endure many of the same requirements except their traditional clients are the pest control industry (exterminators and structural/landscape pesticide manufacturers — basically, the same people who manufacture agrichemicals). However, a number of black sheep out there are taking the huge risk of providing information and services to non-traditional audiences.

Specifically, they see the school community as a client. A few are diverting some of the time they normally would spend responding to the pest control industry to provide training, pesticide efficacy data and fact sheets to develop IPM materials tailored to the school community. They also conduct pilot IPM programs in some school districts. Some get small EPA grants to do so, but a few are doing it simply because it's what they believed they would be doing when they became professionals — and because it is just the "right thing to do". Some of the university entomologists with whom I have worked to implement these non-traditional programs include Tim Gibb, Al Fournier and Fred Whitford in Indiana (partners in starting our Monroe IPM Model programs), Carl Olson and Paul Baker in Arizona and Fudd Graham and Mike Williams in Alabama.. They're fun people, risk takers and damn' good entomologists.

I must pay special deference to Dawn Gouge in Arizona, who as an untenured urban entomology professor and young mother has addressed the good ol' boy system with professional know-how, maternal ferocity and English charm that are changing the system. These black sheep get very little credit for these activities during their annual performance reviews because their administration doesn't recognize them as achieving the missions dictated by the USDA. You need big bucks in grant money to overcome this obstacle, and the USEPA isn't offering it. For sure, the school community isn't.

- Pesticide Manufacturers?

Yes, I am saying that there is and has been some good work from a narrow sector of this group. Unfortunately, the effects of the larger and more powerful sector of this industry give these "Good" folks a bad name (see "The Bad" section). However, it would be unfair not to list some of the good works from good people.

To my knowledge the toxicity of pesticides, particularly structural use insecticides, has decreased considerably in the past 20 years. Thanks to some great science, insecticides have been developed that rely more on the pests' reproductive and feeding behavior, thereby allowing for a safer and more selective kill. Many of these products have been developed from pathogens and chemicals that the Natural World has evolved to compete with specific insects over millennia. These products are typically developed at a cost of approximately one $100 million per product, and someone is making the conscious decision to do that. I have good friends that work for pesticide manufacturers who have done the Research and Development (R&D) for these products, However, they have also worked tirelessly to support IPM specialists in order to better develop and implement substitution of these products for safer or IPM-compatible pesticides. Indeed, I would not feel comfortable demonstrating a real IPM program in a pest-infested school system if I could not rely on the occasional and very selective use of these IPM tools.

Alas, much like some antibiotics — that once were lifesaving tools in the medical profession but now are no longer useful, or worse, through their misuse have allowed even worse super- (resistant) bacteria to eat our flesh and ravage our bodies — these new pesticides many have worked so hard to develop are becoming useless. Why? Because of greed and the bottom line. Historically, companies that induce patients to request new (and expensive) drugs, and give doctors incentives to over-proscribe those same drugs, are the same manufacturers (though their names and/ or ownership have changed) that induce farmers and homeowners and their pest management professionals to over-use these valuable pesticides. It's back to the old pesticide snowball effect. For the great scientists who brought us these silver bullets, no good deed goes unpunished.

The Bad

These are the people who scare the hell out of you so they can take your money. They have convinced you that the only good bug is a dead bug, that you are a bad neighbor if you have dandelions and that you can't pull weeds: you must spray them. Your home is at risk, as is your life. They are the same industry groups that consistently and relentlessly attacked Rachael Carson for writing *Silent Spring* and call themselves "green ...red, white and blue". Compare their propaganda from the mid-'60s to present — there is not a whole lot of difference. They are the folks who have donated to enough political campaigns that they have produced elected officials who chant, "based on sound science" and "we need more studies". Those mantra ensure that they don't have to take meaningful action to protect our citizens and steward our earth.

Chemical pesticides and the people who apply them are valuable and, at times, necessary tools for managing pests. Yes, they can save lives and our homes. Bless the researchers and the company dollars that develop them. The problem is the quarterly report that shows the bottom line and the folks who never can have enough. They are greedy "liars, damn' liars and statisticians" (Disraeli).

- Pesticide Manufacturers

How could anybody or any institution be against protecting children from unnecessary exposure to and the unneeded expense of pesticides in schools and daycare facilities? Well, according to RISE® (Responsible Industry for a Sound Environment) and CropLife America (formerly the American Crop Protection Association), *they* certainly are not. Horse pucky! These are the same lobbying organizations (under different names) that ruthlessly attacked Rachael Carson during the publication of her book, and spent millions developing anti-*Silent Spring* propaganda from the time of its publication into the 1970s. It's their job! These associations are pesticide manufacturing industry lobbying groups. RISE® works the structural/landscape pesticide side of the industry and CropLife works the agricultural side. Many companies belong to both organizations. They're dedicated to breaking down any barriers their membership might encounter in selling pesticides. And they are very good at it — much better than they were in the late 60s in responding to *Silent Spring*. For those of you young enough to remember, the messages were very similar — except for insinuating that anti-pesticide folks were communists. Rush Limbaugh ranted, "Elimination of dangerous pesticides is a conspiracy by liberals". He was referring to controversy about balancing the use of pesticides, grapes and black widow spiders (Pruess, 2003). Yeah, who needs communists when you have liberals.

RISE® and CropLife send out mom, the flag and apple pie messages that are designed to make a person feel ignorant or unpatriotic if he/she disagrees with, "Rats, cockroaches, stinging insects and other pests seriously threaten the health and safety of our children and all citizens"; "Pesticides are thoroughly tested, well regulated, safely used and effectively monitored"; "It's the Law: IPM Includes the Use of 'Chemical Tools'"; "IPM has consistently and enthusiastically been supported by the pesticide industry" (RISE® Fact Sheets, 2002). RISE® and CropLife try to convince the public that pesticides provide health and lifestyle benefits derived from lush, green lawns — in ads underwritten by Project Evergreen — another trade association made up of pesticide makers, applicators, garden centers and mower manufacturers (Lowy, 2005).

Heaven forbid that our children and all citizens should be seriously threatened by "Rats, cockroaches, stinging insects and other pests", or be deprived of picture-perfect lawns. Don't you believe that our government makes sure that pesticides are regulated properly? You can be damn' sure that RISE® and CropLife support IPM with all the right buzz words, programs and awards. But nearly all of it is half truths, as you will soon read.

I said it before and I say it now — pesticides are an important tool for pest management. However, you and your children are not seriously threatened by pests to the extent that warrants the amounts of pesticides (individually or through exterminators) you are told to purchase and use. This unnecessary use is in large part due to the fear tactics used by this very industry to promote pesticide use. Further, pesticides are not well regulated. We have well-meaning USEPA, State Lead Agency and Cooperative Extension personnel who are trying their best to regulate and educate for the best use of pesticides. But have you scrutinized their budgets lately? They are under-funded or unfunded in their mandates to protect us from improper pesticide registration and application. A long time ago, former Comptroller of the Pentagon General Frank Sackton told me that agency programs are not a priority unless they have an adequate budget.

The fact is that these hired guns have taken away the power of local public officials to legally limit pesticide use in recent years. They have lobbied state legislatures to pass pre-emption laws, that provide the states authority for pesticide regulation, and they prevent cities and towns from enacting their own laws. "Local communities generally do not have the expertise on issues about pesticides to make responsible decisions...[these decisions] are made much more carefully and the train moves much more slowly at the state level," said Allen James, president of RISE® (Lowy, 2005).

Please ask your congressional representatives where they get their information about how to spend federal and state money on pesticide programs. Ask Congressman Tom Delay of Texas, former owner of a pest control business, who still believes DDT should not have been banned (Perl, 2001), where he gets his information and what campaign contributions he gets from RISE® partners. These folks have much deeper pockets than Beyond Pesticides or other groups and lots of power in their hired guns. That fact no doubt will be pointed out to me after this book comes out — it won't be the first time. But, I forget, why should I fear any association that "consistently and enthusiastically" supports IPM? Sure.

What is the support of IPM to which these industry support groups profess? They did distribute the famous *Pest Control in the School Environment: Adopting Integrated Pest Management* (affectionately known as the "Rat Book") that the USEPA put out about IPM in schools (USEPA, 1993). I admit it's a decent piece of work. Of course, it is my understanding from Ralph Wright and Bill Curry, both former Office of Pesticide Program officials, that RISE® spent literally years of lobbying to get this book published in a more-pesticide-dependent version than early drafts. RISE® sponsors an awards program through Texas A&M's Southwest School Technical Resource Center — $1,000 and $500 awards to schools that fill out questionnaires crafted, in part by RISE®.

Perhaps another example of its "support" for reducing unnecessary pesticide exposure to children would be the "inside the beltway" RISE® response to the Zahm and Ward article, *Pesticides and Childhood Cancer*, submitted to *Environmental Health Perspectives* in 1997 (Zahm & Devesa, 1995). RISE® accused the authors of making "inflammatory and unsubstantiated statements" because "As there are non-conclusive scientific findings that pesticides cause cancer in children, there is no scientific support for the concept that reduced exposures to pesticides would lead to a reduction in cancer risk" (RISE®, 1998). The "let's have better science" and "more studies" arguments from RISE® subverted Zahm's and Ward's compelling argument that children were exposed to many potentially harmful pesticides from multiple sources (Zahm & Devesa, 1995, Goldman, 1995, Eskenazi, et.al.,1999). How 'bout RISE®'s duplicitous support for the 2002 School Environmental Protection Act (SEPA) where, somehow, the Senate Agriculture Committee was prompted into deciding that the House Education Committee did not have jurisdiction to vote on an IPM mandate for schools? The bill has yet to be heard. Or more recently, the July, 2002, joint letter to Stephen Johnson, then Assistant Administrator for the Office of Pesticide Programs? The letter requested his intervention, protesting the invitation of Dr. Lynn Goldman, Dr. Philip Landrigan and Dr. Richard Jackson (three nationally recognized experts) to participate in the "National Strategies for Health Care Providers: Pesticides Initiative" forum for training healthcare workers in the prevention of pesticide poisonings and exposures (US Congress, 2002,). This USEPA-funded forum was postponed. Hey, it's the job of the lobbying hired gun to kill the opposition, but it is difficult to hear of RISE's actions as "consistent and enthusiastic support" without feeling like they are blowing in my ear.

The examples above, though egregious in my opinion, are at least straightforward examples of not really "consistently and enthusiastically" supporting IPM. However, a far darker contribution by the industry is the fashion in which it subverts its messages of support. This is done in two ways: One I touched on earlier when discussing the subtle and not-so-subtle co-optation of regulatory and educational professionals. The other involves the role of salesman versus technical, research and development representatives.

We all love to be appreciated. It's human nature. Most scientists who work for universities, and especially government agencies, are under-appreciated and/or underpaid. So when we are invited to speak to or participate with our colleagues on a national or international level, at classy resorts and/or conference centers, expenses paid, we feel appreciated. I'm talking about places we normally couldn't afford to visit, doing things we couldn't afford to do on little side trips (golf, fishing, hunting, etc.) and interacting with folks who act as though they really want to hear what we are saying. Think about it. While attending my first Entomological Society of America meeting as a grad student I discovered the wonders of hospitality suites — delicious little food items on elegant platters, free booze and trinkets (caps, pocketknives, pens) — all the things that poor grad students need in order to feel good about what they are doing. And don't get me wrong: the pesticide companies footing the bill weren't asking me to do anything wrong — just be appreciated.

This appreciation became an entitlement. Our mentoring professors were there and it was okay. It was legal for government officials. No money, no favors, and why not? It's not like the public was treating us that well. In truth, we really did learn quite a bit from the networking that was provided. I am not saying this was all wrong...just one-sided.

Many of us were attempting to implement IPM or regulate pesticides and by God, this was where the pesticide makers were consistently and enthusiastically supporting us. The folks I was exposed to weren't poison peddlers. They were guys like me performing R&D for multinational companies and advising people how to use their "tools" in a manner consistent with IPM. What they said made scientific sense and I believed them. They believed themselves. The only trouble was the bottom line. That decision to commit $100 million to develop a new pesticide product had an even larger price.

Over the last 20-some years, I have attended many, many professional conferences – mostly ones conducted by the Entomological Society of America. This is a wonderful professional society that has enriched my life immensely in terms of scientific knowledge and great friendships. Of course, several thousand extremely good-looking entomologists who get excited about playing with bugs, also constitutes a very stimulating venue. Drop in on one of our conferences some time. While many of the papers presented deal with the study of insects and their relatives (ecology, physiology, pathology, taxonomy, etc.), most of the presentations I have attended involved managing these animals in their competition with humans — pest management. These papers usually are presented by university entomologists under industry-sponsored research (pesticide manufacturers pay you to conduct research on their products) and/or by pesticide manufacturer employees (research or technical representatives). I have presented a number of papers, as I have conducted many field trials on the effectiveness of new or about-to-be-registered insecticides. During these presentations I began to ask myself, "How can these company reps keep saying they believe in IPM and resistance management and at the same time consistently tout the 'broad spectrum' effectiveness of their insecticides? Or, that their product has 'better residual control' than that of their competitors? In other words, they said they believed that natural enemies (good bugs) are vital to an IPM approach, but that their product was superior because it killed bugs other than the target pest. And they contended that environmentally persistent insecticides are better because they kill longer. This approach has not changed in the years I have been attending such presentations. Is this consistent support of real IPM? While some of my colleagues might argue with me regarding a few specific applications, I don't think so.

By addressing where the bottom line meets the consumer — sales —I end my explanation of how pesticide manufacturers subvert attempts to reduce use of unnecessary pesticides. I am not against making money (I hope you bought this book!), but the bottom line is that manufacturers must recoup their investments and satisfy their stockholders. I would hope they do this by selling a product that is truly needed. The lies begin when the product is sold but not needed. Look at their advertising. By far, the greatest reduction of pesticide use I demonstrate in my programs is from simply saying, "Stop applying pesticides until you know you have a problem!" Just who is telling exterminators, school officials and you that there is a reason to use pesticides, and how do they do it? Pesticides don't prevent pests any more than antibiotics prevent bacteria, but the advertisement or sales reps say so! Phrases like "at the first sign of...", and "provides the best insurance for..." are rife in industry advertisements. My industry R&D friends cringe at how their company sales people misrepresent products. The lies continue when the product is sold as doing something it doesn't. Why do exterminators spray for lice when it doesn't work? Where in the advertising is the consistent and enthusiastic support for using chemical pesticides only when necessary (IPM)? Read it in the aisles of your supermarket or your hardware store, or on company websites. Ask your exterminator for product pamphlets, ads on TV, or attend the annual Pest Management Conference offered by your state lead agency and/or Cooperative Extension and just listen to the sales reps. For you folks who always drive the speed limit: The fact that "the use of 'chemical tools'" is included in the legal definition of IPM doesn't mean you HAVE to use chemicals. And, the ultimate lie is, "Trust us".

- Exterminators

Notice I say Exterminators. Unfortunately, some real Pest Management Professionals (PMPs) are forced to wear patches that say Exterminator. Make no mistake; I am not talking about Pest Management Professionals who are well trained, keep up with their professional education and adhere to ethical standards. I am talking about folks more concerned with selling a pesticide application service and quickly moving to the next "account", who are not well trained, don't keep up with their professional education and don't necessarily adhere to ethical standards — exterminators. Is that sufficiently black and white? "Red Flags" that indicate an exterminator rather than a Pest Management Professional is at your door:

1) They first come to your facility carrying a spray can;
2) They don't carry or use a flashlight and notebook;
3) They can't (won't) tell you the name and/or active ingredients of the pesticides they are using;
4) They don't take the time to point out conducive conditions or give you instructions for their remediation; and
5) They are working under their manager's Pest Control Operator license.

I have discussed these guys a bit already in terms of scaring the hell out of people so they can take their money. A lot of problems with the pesticide manufacturing industry apply equally to the exterminator segment of the pest control industry. However, these folks commit particularly evil deeds.

Most Pest Management Professionals I know can't stand the guys who work out of the back of their car. They cannot abide their lack of professionalism and they can't compete with the low bids these folks offer and are awarded, from under-budgeted schools. The worst of these folk are those who use the phrase IPM and have no idea how to implement it or are too cheap to implement it. Of course, that's where this book comes in — now you know what to ask. I know of non-licensed operators who sprayed restricted agricultural chemicals (called "roach milk" because of its appearance in solution, and packaged in used milk containers) throughout homes of pre-schoolers. They also sprayed banned insecticides in air ducts. I meet exterminators who can't tell a fruit fly from a moth fly, a pavement ant from a fire ant — all of which have different conducive conditions for becoming pests and different methods to control them. These guys apply pesticides illegally or incorrectly, don't have the know-how or equipment to monitor for pest activity, can't recognize conducive conditions, communicate only to sell their services and, worse, give schools and parents a false sense of security — at taxpayer expense. Maggots!

The worst group is the slick salesmen with a good hefty budget. They are licensed and trained, but sales volume is the name of the game. How many contracts per sales area can they get, what kind of "call-back for extra service" rate do they have, and how can they reduce expenses by not honoring warrantees, hiring unskilled workers at minimum wage, diluting pesticides, not monitoring or not taking the time to educate their customers about conducive conditions? Many of these people have names on the stock exchange. What is so bad is that they know what IPM is and have made the conscious decision to market it, but not use it. It just isn't profitable...enough.

What usually happens when I begin working with a school district that contract with the likes of these folks is the "exterminators" piss and moan about how they already are practicing IPM. Then they disappear (kinda like roaches into the woodwork?). PMPs, while not always welcoming, usually cooperate, tag along, sometimes lead and often end up teaching me as much as I do them. Meanwhile, the exterminators complain they are losing their contract, start rumors about how the "IPM Program" is failing, and go to their state exterminator associations and start movements against government/university school IPM programs.

These we-are-gonna-lose-our-livelihoods-if-schools-opt-for-IPM movements have been pretty successful in many states where I have worked. Of course, some of my colleagues say it's just Marc's sterling personality that drives these folks to such desperate measures. My number one school administrator pal, John Carter, when presenting the results of the Monroe County Community School Corporation IPM program at an Entomological Society Meeting in 1996, said of exterminators in his school district, "The first thing we did was kick them out!" Bobby Corrigan and Tim Gibb still roll their eyes at the memory — mine just tear up with laughter. Well, it hit the fan after that cute remark. Bobby had to spend extra time explaining who the hell he was working with; Tim's department head at Purdue was asked by the pest control industry reps to "speak" to him; and I didn't get a baseball cap from any exterminator companies that year. Seriously, all this happened — except I really wasn't expecting a cap. There are state training programs for IPM in schools that I have not been allowed to participate in, or I have been taken off the agenda of such programs once people subject to pressures from the pest control industry got word of my attendance. Industry grants to participating entomologists have been threatened if those professionals pushed the professional standards and ethics issue too far. Fortunately, this segment of the pest control industry has such a bad reputation most people who make contract decisions for school districts are not harassed to a great degree. That's not the case with their traditional service providers in Cooperative Extension and State Lead Agencies.

Though I find the National Pest Management Association's efforts to develop training and standards for those practicing IPM in schools to be sorely lacking, in many other ways it seems to be addressing those who wish to become Professional Pest Managers in this country. This is a supply-side effort aimed at transitioning/professionalizing folks who might have been exterminators, but who recognize the value of implementing IPM. This effort will be for naught unless school system decisionmakers are convinced to (or allowed to) address the demand side of IPM in partnership with PMPs. And the first step is for them to understand "The Bad" they currently are dealing with.

- Farmer Associations and the Farm Press

For reasons of money and maintaining power, agricultural producer and lawn-care industry lobbying groups (and their trade journals that advertise agrichemicals) feel it necessary to demonize environmentalists of any stripe. This really burns me, as I am a big fan of the American farmer and consciously sought a career working with farmers. While I see

57

the majority of farmers as true conservationists and stewards of the land, they seem to hate the word environmentalist. When you want to get a rise out of them, just connote environmentalist and they get riled.

The industry began using the term anti-pesticide to mean anti-farmer when *Silent Spring* came out (even though Carson was not anti-pesticide, but anti the unnecessary use of pesticides), and it worked well – still does. Remember that many of our elected representatives in Washington, D.C. feel the need to keep agriculture happy. Consequently, outfits like the Farm Bureau and the like are still working that power base. Their testimony to the House or Senate Agricultural Committees, or their public comments regarding rules and regulations promoting IPM, are in the public record. Lately, the attack has become more focused on school IPM.

In a recent commentary, Harry Cline of the Western Farm Press wrote on behalf of Allen James, president of RISE®, that school administrators in several states are desperate because they can no longer use pesticides. He said further that anti-pesticide advocacy groups are using schools to further their cause… that they refuse to work with industry, that pesticides are critical for the health of our children, and so he urged farmers, "Talk to your local school administrators and tell them you support pesticide use". The rationale for his patriotic rally cry was, "because it is a battle agriculture must join to ensure victory" (Cline, 2001). Some Extension IPM specialists who wanted to respond but were concerned for their job security urged me to do so. This was my reply:

Dear Mr. Cline,

As an individual who spent a significant portion of my life living and working in the southwestern farming community I found your commentary of November 3 ("School anti-pesticide drive is everyone's fight in nation") rather disturbing. I work with school districts all over the US to better manage their pests. Better management means reduced risks to children and reduced costs to tax payers. I am NOT anti-pesticide, but I am against the unnecessary use of pesticides. Every school district that I have worked with had applied pesticides on a scheduled basis, and there was virtually no consultation between pest management professionals regarding pest management practices (what products for what problems and more effective alternatives). Would a progressive farmer use such a "hands off" management strategy? This current, traditional approach to pest management in those schools resulted in a gross overuse of pesticides and a less than adequate reduction of pest problems. Perhaps more important, school administrators were unaware of what practices were employed, as was the rest of the school community.

Mr. Cline, children are not crops and farmers know it. You are grossly misinformed, or worse, a shill for the pesticide industry – maybe both. Fact, the states you mentioned (as well as others) require some parental notification prior to some pesticide application, recommend low impact options to be used IF available and exempt almost all registered pesticides for emergency public health conditions in or around schools. This is something I, as a taxpayer, applaud – better management. Fact, RISE has not tried to work with schools or concerned citizens except to produce fact sheets and send form letters to school officials portraying all pests as dangerous and pesticides as a critical and recommended panacea. Any attribution to IPM is in words only with no attempt to explain the critical nature of communication or partnership required for the successful implementation of this concept. Further, there has been no attempt by RISE to recognize that pesticides might be used unnecessarily or exacerbate rather than remedy a pest situation – something farmers have long battled in the form of insecticide resistance. Fact, the movement of local and state government to assist and/or mandate school districts to implement best management practices (including IPM and the "right to know" for community members regarding pesticide use) not only is responsible to the tax payer but also represents the best in modern public health practices.

Perhaps instead of asking farmers to "Talk to your local school administrators and tell them you support pesticide use", you might ask farmers to urge school districts to implement a verifiable IPM program, and even offer assistance regarding what real IPM is (including chemical use when monitoring indicates and other controls fail). I for one know that the American farmer has lots to offer our children and their schools. Further, they have been blamed far too much by uninformed citizens and DO NOT need to become shills for the pesticide industry. [Lame (in Cline), 2001]

Now, I believe I have met Harry Cline at farm meetings in Arizona over the years, and he always impressed me as a pretty nice guy. Why did he feel the need to rally the agricultural community against school IPM? Could it be that while RISE® was professing support for the proposed

School Environmental Protection Act, it was working the other side of the fence (influencing folks who use and advertise their members' pesticide products) to develop support against this act? As I mentioned before, the act was moved from the House Education Committee to the Senate Agriculture Committee and never heard.

The Ugly

While I certainly believe that Bad entities have some fear of IPM, they are motivated mostly by greed. Not so this next group. This is us — our public servants. Yes, there are greedy "empire builders" in this group, but for the most part, they are afraid. They stonewall you, and flat won't do their jobs. They are afraid of losing their jobs, power, territory and prestige. Once you recognize it, you can see the fear in their eyes, and it is Ugly.

- Our Schools

The last thing I expected when I began to implement IPM in schools was that one group that would consistently resist this implementation would be the school administrators (particularly their lobbyist groups). It is my experience that about one third of school principals could care less about pests or pesticides as long as they don't have parents or teachers complaining about bugs in the school or dandelions around the flagpole. Most principals have standardized tests, drug abuse, suicide, homicide, burned-out teachers, pushy parents, pushier coaches and on and on to deal with. Many teachers are in the same boat. However, most of these "site-based managers" are willing to go along so long as IPM is not an additional item on their plate. And really good IPM programs are not.

Our problem surfaces when we have a school superintendent who will not make decisions on this issue, or when the school facilities and/or food service managers are petty bureaucrats. They are AFRAID of change. Many of these people (and I can sympathize with them to some extent) worked their way up through the system, attained management positions when the school system was smaller and now are overwhelmed by the size and scope of their job. Any new responsibility is a threat that can make them look bad, make someone else look better or add to their workload. The standard way they cope with the size and scope is to contract out services they understand to people who promise they can keep others from complaining. Look at the pest control contracts your school district has. Were they obtained under "requests for proposal" (lowest bids) or "requests for qualifications" (abilities — which is far better)? What oversight is involved? Why is pest management a contracted function in your school district? Is it because the school facilities and/or kitchen manager doesn't have the budget or willing staff who could internalize pest management (as was done with Jerry Jochim in Bloomington, Indiana, and the Kyrene School District in Tempe, Arizona)? Is the school district happy with the contractor it has? Or perhaps they don't want to go through the bid process for pest management, or just don't want to be responsible for these program functions? John Carter at Monroe County-Community School Corporation will tell you that his management pertaining to building health and safety has become easier since he went to IPM, but John is a pro who is not afraid of change. In fact, John embraces change as part of good management. Embrace versus fear.

Another reason school administrations (according to the testimony of their state and national associations) have resisted the mandatory notification of pesticide application is that it will cost too much in staff time and materials. What horse pucky! First, the school community has the right to know if it is being exposed to a potentially hazardous product. Yes, it will cost more to notify the community if these types of products are used. That's the point! John testified to the Indiana State House Education Committee when confronted with this supposed tale of woe. He stated simply that, "Using IPM costs less in staff time and materials, not only because we just don't use materials that require public notification, but also because we don't have to spend time on parent and staff complaints about pests and pesticides". So, what's the problem? Too much change and not enough competence and guts, as you will later read about the Clark County (Las Vegas) School District. Of course, this is why it is particularly important for parents and/or child advocacy groups to get involved in facilitating change, as Tom Neltner (IKE) did in the Indianapolis Public Schools. The best place to start is by arranging a meeting with the school superintendent, your Cooperative Extension IPM Specialist and your State Lead Agency. Aren't they there to protect and educate?

- Our Protectors (regulators and activists)

Unfortunately, since the Congressional Revolution of 1994, spending for environmental and children's health programs has suffered at the federal level. Elected representatives who believe environmental laws are too onerous and/or that pesticides are God's gift to our species are not about to vote against them. They just deny funding needed to implement them so regulators can't do their jobs. Mandated programs are unfunded or under-funded. Spending goes down and pesticide manufacturing industry influence goes up. Not only have those regulators who believe IPM is the way to reduce pesticide exposure to children (thereby complying with the intent of FIFRA and the Food Quality Protection Act) been hobbled by the budgetary process, but they have also become targets of the hired guns from the pesticide and pest management industry. All it takes is a letter to a division head or higher expressing "concern" over agency actions to stop promoters of IPM dead in their tracks. I am sorry to say that people I do like and respect have caved in upon receipt of such messages, and who can blame them? I have witnessed this with the USEPA, USDA and even the GAO when they had the audacity to investigate what the government was doing about pesticides in schools or the lack of the national implementation of IPM (GAO, 1999 and 2001). It is no wonder that, in an environment of intimidation and very limited resources, our regulatory protectors are turf-bound and afraid to be reasonably aggressive and innovative. Ask your Congressmen or senator why there is no budgetary line item for IPM in schools and why, after 10 years of demonstrating that IPM can reduce pests and pesticides in the school environment, there is no comprehensive national strategy to diffuse IPM in schools throughout the U.S.

Combine this environment with the culture of agricultural agencies in the U.S, and the uphill climb for IPM becomes even steeper. Agency culture? Sounds like I teach public administration, and I do. Who are the entities that implement pest management programs or regulate pesticides for states and the USDA, and what is their mission? In general, the mission of agricultural agencies in the U.S. is to protect and promote agri-business. This includes industries that produce agricultural commodities, farm machinery and agrichemicals. Their mission has not been to protect human health and the environment. That is the mission of other agencies, and I am okay with that — unless the USDA presumes to take on the mission of protecting human health and the environment in an incompetent manner or, worse, stalls. Most of the people who work for agricultural agencies are white men with agricultural backgrounds, and they have become very good at making (and keeping) the U.S. the best country in the world at providing food and fiber — and agri-business. Too many of these guys (excluding more heroic types like Carl Martin, Larry Swain, Chuck Moses and others in many states) still buy into the myth that pesticides are saving our planet (Avery, 2000), and most view their clientele as pesticide users — that's peer comfort. In 2002, colleagues of mine were asked by their State Lead Agency not to have me work on implementing IPM in Ohio schools. It seems their state's pest control industry association did not want any model programs or outspoken troublemakers. Indeed, I did not visit Ohio until the State Lead Agency administration changed. By the way, we just completed a very successful Monroe IPM Model program near Columbus.

From a regulatory point of view, the problem is that entities (pesticide manufacturers, pest control advisors, pesticide applicators and pest control operators), who are supposed to be regulated, are the same entities that are supposed to be protected and promoted. What we have is a conflict of missions. State Lead Agencies are supposed to enforce FIFRA regulations, but usually are part of the state agricultural agency. Attend a pesticide review board meeting at your state agricultural department or a structural pest control board meeting. Shut-up and observe:

- the proceedings of the meeting;
- the discussions among individuals before the meeting; during breaks and after the meeting;
- who is in the audience; and
- what level of action is taken against any regulatory violation.

Tell me I am wrong, but I have attended these types of meetings for more than 20 years and very little has changed. I hate to say it, because many of these folks I call friends, but it is a good ol' boy system, and pretty Ugly when it comes to "doing the right thing".

I want to conclude our Ugly Protector section by discussing "shoot from the lip activists". I believe I have made it very clear how much I believe activists must be part of this system. However, some of the tactics applied by the hired guns from industry are also used by the activist community, and they scare the hell out of well-meaning regulators. Many times regulators deserve harsh reviews, but try communicating with them first. Above all, make sure you know what you are talking about. I must tell you the opposition does have the elements of its battle plan carefully aligned. It has funding to research the issues and its own preconceived ideas of which scientific and legal solutions regulators and educators should use. For these reasons, regulators and educators view industry as more credible — even if they would really rather help out the public activist. I experienced this as a Cooperative Extension educator and as a state environmental official. Most regulators I know who do want to "do the right thing" will help activists (since activists are part of their public clientele it can be considered within the scope of their job), learn how the system works and what is needed to make it work their way (O'leary, 1994). Then, if your patient communication efforts don't work, eat their ugly spleens.

- Our Educators

Whoa, I have to be careful on this. I do think of myself as an educator. I do teach courses in Management Communications, Environmental Management, Public Management and Insects and the Environment to graduate and undergraduate students. I try to be a good advisor to students regarding their courses of study and the many environmental internships available to them. Most of my work implementing IPM in schools is as an educator (although I love crawling around under dishwashers in school cafeterias looking for bugs). As ombudsman for the Arizona Department of Environmental Quality I was an educator helping regulated entities and the public negotiate their way through our system. But before all this I was an Extension educator with the University of Arizona's Department of Entomology as an IPM Specialist. I seldom thought of myself as ugly, but I learned that sometimes the system is.

As I have mentioned, the system that provides education about pest management for farmers, farm workers who apply pesticides, pesticide manufacturers, agricultural pest control advisors and their urban counterparts (the structural and landscape pest control operators) is the Land Grant University Cooperative Extension system. We called it the Agricultural Extension Service, way back when. As part of the USDA, Cooperative Extension assisted in protecting and promoting agriculture with its applied field research and extension of those solutions to the agriculture community. Most Extension Agents and Specialists had the same background: rural, white males, educated at a Land Grant University School of Agriculture. Every state has one (though now under different school names such as School Agriculture and the Environment, or Ag and Natural Resources). Some southern states have two — a leftover from the segregation days. Auburn University and Tuskegee University are an example. Many of us grew up in this system: 4-H, Ag School, then County Agent or Extension Specialist. We believed. I still believe that Extension is one of the best institutions ever to happen to this country and to the world. Our lives would not be the same if we didn't have a system to bring the knowledge from the university to the farmer who can't come to the university. Our Peace Corps is based on the same model. For Extension entomologists it all worked great until Rachael came along, crops failed because of resistant insect attacks and entomologists like Perry Adkisson (Arkansas) and Robert Van den Bosh (California) developed a crop protection system which later would be called IPM. Then things got ugly.

Remember, organizations that extended pest management practices through research, demonstration of new technologies (mostly pesticides) and information dissemination had their traditional customers (pesticide users) and supporters (pesticide manufacturers) pretty much feeling like they were doing "good" — "better living through chemistry". I remember writing newsletters and fact sheets and conducting workshops that featured all the new pesticides. Farmers described what they wanted and industry described what it had available. Both groups sat on university boards and/ or contributed heavily to the schools of agriculture.

In Arizona IPM was passed off with a wink and a nod by the most powerful farmers and industry. Right before I was hired, my bosses and mentors at the university, Drs. Leon Moore and Theo Watson (known to many as the "Theon" twins), who were two of the founding fathers of cotton IPM, along with George Ware refused to continue to recommend DDT-Toxaphene for cotton insect pest management. Instead, they strongly suggested maybe farmers should have a shorter growing season (lower yields of cotton, but with much lower inputs or cost – better for the farmer and the environment). These tactics landed them in hot water. How could they not recommend what was considered the backbone of the pesticide arsenal at the time? Worse, how could they possibly deprive the agrichemical industry of long season cotton revenue? Immediately, calls for their dismissal assailed the University. Fortunately, they survived (barely, as Dr. George Ware tells it), but the battle lines were drawn throughout the country (Ware, 1994). Van den Bosh and others were attacked, research monies dried up for, or in some cases were supplied to shut up, entomologists who were attempting to extend IPM to farmers (Van den Bosh, 1978). In the university system, tenure can help protect you from administrations that are pressured to fire professors but heaven help the untenured.

I was the "Theon" twins' "pit bull" and, of course, didn't have tenure — yet. As mentioned in chapter one, I learned early what was expected of me and tried to please. I loved my job. Leon's best advice to me (which I often pass on) is, "The best way to learn and do this job right is to 'get your hands dirty'". What's not to love? Working outdoors with bugs and helping the American farmer. While the majority of folks I worked with weren't really receptive to IPM (central Arizona cotton lands were called "Fort Apache" by some IPM folks — as in dangerous territory), we figured that a window of opportunity to implement IPM would open sometime. It did when the boll weevil invaded Arizona cotton. The use and cost of pesticides to control this historical scourge of cotton nearly tripled.

We developed and implemented an area-wide IPM program for boll weevils (and other cotton pests) in the community of Laveen, which was the hotbed of the infestation. We got all farmers in the area to cooperate, and within a year we drastically reduced pesticide use and damage from pests. In the meantime, the USDA's Animal Plant Health Inspection Service (APHIS) was implementing a more pesticide-based eradication program in the Carolinas. This program was subsidized by the government, thereby costing farmers less. Cotton grower associations throughout the country love those subsidies. They soon took over our program, and began experiencing secondary pest (beet armyworm) problems, which required even more pesticide use. Although I had been warned by the Extension administration not to upset APHIS, I sent out a newsletter to cotton growers which documented that the armyworm outbreak was probably an effect of Malathion being used to control the boll weevil. And the proverbial poop hit the fan.

The USDA does not brook interference when conducting eradication programs. In fact they were mightily upset when Carson exposed the effects of their Red Imported Fire Ant Eradication program in the early '60s. Most entomologists now agree that, unless circumstances are absolutely right, eradication programs don't work. I knew I was in trouble when the leader of Arizona's Cotton Grower's Association called my office and said he was going to have me fired. Though I had heard that APHIS and the Cotton Grower's Association had warned the university not to cause any problems, I figured I was just doing my job disseminating field data — and that I had protection under academic freedom. As I look back, I realize I should have waited. I was pragmatic and naïve. Within weeks I was relegated to identifying crickets in a small office and several months later was informed I would be terminated. Maybe if I had waited six months to send out the newsletter? My promotion and tenure package had just been approved by my department and was on its way to be confirmed by the college dean (usually a pro-forma action). Without explanation, the College denied my tenure. In the university system, untenured faculty who are not confirmed by their college receive a "terminal contract". Thus, my career as an Extension IPM Specialist was ended.

To my everlasting appreciation, university entomologists throughout the Cotton Belt (North Carolina to California) tried, in vain, to save me. I received a job offer from the state of North Carolina to run a pest management program, but it was mysteriously taken back days later with no explanation. Friends and foe all knew that extreme pressure had been applied to terminate and blackball me. This later was documented, and I received a settlement offer. These unconscionable tactics have been applied to many vulnerable implementers of IPM by greedy and/or scared organizations. Fortunately, most of those implementers pulled back in time to save themselves, but you can bet those smear tactics slowed down or stopped the implementation of IPM.

The good news for me was that the governor of Arizona needed a person to deal with some hot environmental issues. Since I had a regular TV spot in which I discussed agricultural issues and IPM, I had earned some credibility with the environmental community. I became a troubleshooter for the Arizona Department of Environmental Quality where I received some great post-graduate experience in how to survive in politics. Better yet, the experience taught me that pressure works both ways, and citizen activists can do things scientists can't. As a true missionary, I never lost my early beliefs, and I retained an evangelical zeal for getting folks to use IPM. I now know that, as an entomologist, most Extension IPM staff are woefully inadequate and therefore ugly in their abilities to overcome, rather than hide from, political situations – not to mention develop political support through the inclusion of the non-university, non-agribusiness community.

Inclusion? Perhaps one of the ugliest problems Extension has is that many of its IPM Specialists feel they own IPM. After all, they developed and first demonstrated IPM. The agribusiness people are smart enough to let them believe they own IPM and, as mentioned earlier, agribusinesses are viewed as more credible partners than the average citizen. However, when it comes to school or urban IPM, the citizen or school community becomes the partner, and to exclude them in the effort to implement an IPM program is plain arrogant. Stupid might be the better word. Why wouldn't a salesperson try to relate to his/her customer? I witnessed this communication problem between tech folks and the public when I was with the environmental agency. Is it arrogance or ignorance? Either way, IPM specialists will fail to implement IPM if they don't play nice with their non-scientific partners.

In 1998 I moderated the final session in the first National Workshop for School IPM. Attendees trying to implement school IPM were mostly Extension IPM Specialists. One individual became visibly upset when it was suggested that implementation teams include IPM Specialists, but not be centered at the Land Grant universities, as the best way to implement IPM in schools nationwide. He demanded to know why existing IPM centers created by the USDA should not become the primary implementing entity. I told him it was because Extension was not viewed by the school community as entirely credible and trustworthy. More stuff hit the fan. He and a few of his colleagues were outraged. We all did settle down, but could not come to agreement. Unfortunately, the USEPA, Office of Children's Health Protection, representative at the table became so frightened by this lack of agreement that he recommended his office not support the current direction of IPM. This ugly attitude of "it is my ball and we have to play in my house, my way" cost millions of dollars and years of delay. I have always said that Cooperative Extension should be the leaders, not the owners, when it comes to school IPM. Too bad some don't understand that their entitlement to "own" IPM by agribusiness was gifted and that they must EARN their leadership position with the school community.

- Us

We are not ugly. We are smart — unless we don't make ourselves seen or heard, or if we are ignorant. To me, it is pretty ugly when a parent asks school officials their policy and practices regarding basketball uniforms before they inquire about school security, sanitation and environment. Why? Is it trust in the system, the fear of asking difficult questions or that basketball uniforms are more important? As with many other potentially dangerous or costly problems, we naturally believe bad things can't happen to us and if we do believe they can happen we don't know what to do about it. Pest management is not a high priority with parents or school administrators. I read somewhere in the last few years that in the 1950s, chewing gum was considered one of the major problems in the classroom. Now we have guns and drugs. Thankfully, guns and drugs, while serious, are fairly rare problems, but what about school budgets? Yes, I have made the case that hazardous chemicals and disease are problems (with IPM solutions) that we should care about, but in all fairness how does their occurrence rank compared to lack of monies to teach our children? IPM is good management. It saves money by eliminating unneeded pest control expenses, it enhances building maintenance, and it can prevent the high costs of pesticide or disease exposure and hospitalization. As a taxpayer and parent, I believe it is wrong for school officials not to manage the best for our children and even more wrong if a member of the school community recognizes this without standing up and saying something about it. The fact is, the bad guys wouldn't be getting away with the shenanigans they are if we would just demand better management from our school officials. That is why demand-side IPM is the only way to change the system. The people I discussed in the Bad and Ugly sections of this chapter will change when their customers and public clients demand it. Change is tough and providers will not provide what is needed for real IPM until they are forced to — either politically or from the pocketbook. Believe it or not, I am not asking you to "take to the streets", but I am saying that the school community needs to become informed, to be seen and to be heard. So don't be ugly. Call your school superintendents and if they don't respond

PART III:
Implementation

Chapter Five – "Pest Management is People Management" –Creating the Model for Successful Implementation of IPM in Schools

What I want is for IPM to be adopted by the school community. This means the diffusion of IPM. Diffusion is to a community what adoption is to an individual. In this chapter I will use adoption, diffusion and implementation interchangeably — while knowing they are not exactly the same thing. What is fact (it must be, because I teach it in my Management Communication course — ahem), is that for humans to adopt something new, they must change their behavior, and therefore they need to communicate. Clearly, this communication is needed for the successful implementation of IPM in schools. Currently, communication regarding IPM in schools is relegated to either the pest control industry (which does not view its time spent on communication as reimbursable) or your school administration, which does not consider IPM worth communicating about, and it may not have the expertise to send the proper message(s) about pest management, in any case.

The school IPM model which I introduce in this chapter is based on communication — more specifically, the communication sub-specialty of diffusion. It is my experience that this model for the diffusion of IPM in the school community is the most successful and cost-effective way to protect our children from pests and pesticides. In this chapter you will receive a relatively in-depth exposure to communication science as it relates to diffusion, and you'll be exposed to processes and ideas that were tailor-made for successful diffusion of IPM in schools. Further, you will witness how a model of diffusion for school IPM demonstrated its potential in Bloomington, Indiana.

In his 1995 book *Diffusion of Innovation*, Everett Rogers outlines how the change agent should manage diffusion (Rogers, 1995). As I have mentioned, many of the change agents responsible for implementing IPM (Cooperative Extension, school administrators, pest management professionals, regulators, etc.) have little knowledge of the diffusion process (the process of adoption of an innovation by a community over time). It probably is not necessary that IPM programs be managed by diffusion experts. However, individuals who are managing IPM programs should have knowledge of the diffusion process and access to experts in this field.

Communication 101

There are three basic reasons why one communicates: To give or get information, to affect attitudes and to influence behavior (Garnett, 1992). Communication in the context of implementation relies on skills pertaining to the innovation diffusion process. It is a sub-specialty of communication from which change agents (decisionmakers, senior managers and front-line implementers) can benefit. If one subscribes to Metcalf and Luckmann's writings on influencing people (Metcalf & Luckmann, 1994, p.2) clearly, the benefits of employing diffusion concepts can be manifested in accelerated, successful, IPM program implementation.

According to Rogers (1995, p. 11) an <u>innovation</u> is "... any idea, practice, or object that is perceived as new by an individual or other unit of adoption". Even if such an idea or practice has been around for years, it becomes an innovation if the adopting unit perceives it as new. While <u>diffusion</u> refers to exchange or movement among individuals at a social system level (Lambur et al., 1985), <u>adoption</u> is an act of acceptance or use undertaken by an individual. Two types of diffusion are described by Rogers as centralized and decentralized (Rogers, 1995). A centralized diffusion system is characterized by an element of control. In this setting, issues such as when diffusion starts and identifying the principal channels for dissemination are determined by individuals in a managerial role (e.g., school superintendents) as well as the agency charged with diffusion of an innovation. Decentralized diffusion systems are not characterized as directed change. A major impediment to diffusing IPM in agriculture has been the decentralized nature of the user's communication network (Lame, 1992). However, a major advantage to the centralized nature of public schools is their established and linear communication network.

IPM has some unusual features as an innovation. It is technical, but could also be classified as both a soft innovation and a hard innovation. It is hard in the sense that most technologies that comprise IPM are either concrete procedures (such as pest monitoring or exclusion practices) or products (insecticides, weather-stripping). It is a soft innovation in that it has an intellectual component: IPM in practice is the plan or strategy of implementing the technologies in a coordinated way, using models and policies.

IPM DEFINED AS AN INNOVATION (again)

IPM is a cluster of technologies (cultural, mechanical, biological, genetic and chemical) that is an integrated application (based on biological information) designed to allow humans to compete with other species (pests).

Important subcategories of innovations include Rogers' (1995) five characteristics: relative advantage, compatibility, complexity, trialability and observability. Relative advantage, compatibility, trialability and observability are considered to have a positive effect on diffusion while complexity has a negative effect on the rate of diffusion of an innovation. It is important to look at the properties of the IPM innovation itself to understand how the community might diffuse IPM. In general, the compatibility of IPM with the public school system is excellent as it pertains to education, sanitation, energy conservation and structural maintenance. IPM is very trialable — it can be visually demonstrated. In this context, a three-school trialable pilot program was part of the district IPM implementation plan. The most positive of IPM's attributes is its trialability and observability — affirming for one school district superintendent that his decision to try IPM was right to the extent that he attempted to persuade another superintendent to try IPM. The relative advantage of IPM to schools in the past has not been viewed as an economical alternative to current practices of pest control — it was difficult to demonstrate the economic benefits of IPM over traditional controls. However, when the school district becomes more aware of its environmental health costs, IPM becomes viewed as having distinct relative advantage over traditional controls.

The complexity of the IPM innovation has a definite negative impact on the rate of adoption (Lambur, et al., 1985). IPM is a technology cluster of integrated parts and this integration involves more planning. Further, utilizing technologies within the cluster requires planning more involved than scheduling monthly applications of an insecticide. IPM technologies require knowledge of biology of the insect complex (both pests and beneficials), the timing of special applications and the coordination of management operations (sanitation, maintenance, food preparation and education) to integrate cultural and mechanical controls into one's operation.

The change agents

When we question which entities will affect the behavioral changes necessary for the successful implementation of school IPM, we arrive at the three key actors—local government, management and entomology. Originally, the partnership that implemented the Monroe IPM Model consisted of a local government entity (the school corporation), a program manager (me) contracted by the USEPA, an urban/industrial entomologist from the private sector, an Extension Entomologist and usually a representative from the State Lead Agency. The combination of these entities as change agents has had a synergistic effect on program development and implementation. This has resulted in an innovation or model based not only on the IPM concept, but which also mandates the incorporation of organizational management, policy development and management communication. All partners were initiated by first demonstrating their commitment to a successful IPM program.

In most school districts in the United States the administration structure is highly centralized (a school board, superintendent and principals administrating faculty and staff). The centralized nature of this system is extremely important to implementation of policies and communication within the school community (Rogers, 1993). The administrative decisionmakers (superintendent and assistant superintendent of extended services) examine the results and recommendations of the initial pest management assessment and establish a commitment to the program by moving away from traditional "exterminator" services.

Strategic Planning for IPM Implementation

The change agents for this program agreed to use a technology transfer plan grounded in James Garnett's "strategic planning for communication" innovation. This plan requires describing the management situation/object, the message needed to accomplish the objectives, the audience(s) whose behavior would be influenced, the media tailored to the audience's stage of adoption and a feedback mechanism for program evaluation purposes (Garnett, 1992). This plan was then incorporated into a process described by Rogers (1995) as the Innovation-Decision Process. This process traces or represents a sequence of actions and choices by which individuals or organizations (e.g., an adopting school community) evaluate an innovation to decide whether or not to incorporate it into their management practices (Rogers, 1995). The innovation-decision process has five stages: knowledge, persuasion, decision, implementation and confirmation.

The Management Situation:

The management mission for any IPM change agent is to demonstrate a program that allows schools to more effectively manage their pests while maintaining the safest learning environment. Again, a pest can be defined as an organism that competes with humans for food, water, shelter, or attention. The strategies for successfully competing with pests in the school environment present an unprecedented requirement and opportunity for environmental and behavioral management of the host community. This community consists of administrators, teachers, students, custodial/maintenance staff, kitchen staff, nurses, parent volunteers and pest management contractors. Activities in this environment include education, recreation and the maintenance of human bodily functions (food and water intake and output). This environment and the pests associated with it are basically uniform nationwide.

The Message:

The IPM approach can be successful in the school environment because cultural and mechanical strategies can be incorporated into existing custodial and maintenance activities such as sanitation, energy conservation, building security and infrastructure maintenance. Further, monitoring efficiency is enhanced via the virtual full-time presence and perception of the host community. This strategy depends on an educational approach that can create an awareness by all occupants of a proactive management strategy versus the reactive strategy of chemical treatment. Thus, by incorporating IPM into existing school operations (sanitation, maintenance and classroom education) rather than adding pest control currently performed by contractors, school districts will be able to overcome their natural resistance to adding pest management to an already full plate.

Primary - Integrated Pest Management will allow your school to reduce the number of pests while using fewer potentially harmful pesticides, and you can do so without significantly increasing your current job responsibilities.

Supportive Secondary(s) – Nationwide, most school districts that have successfully implemented IPM say they did so because "it was the right thing to do".

The vast majority of what will be asked of you involves incorporating the knowledge of 'what our pests are and why we have pests' into your existing job responsibilities of facility/food sanitation, energy conservation, building security and education.

Tools you will learn and use to prevent pests in your schools will also work for your home.

The Audience(s):

As discussed earlier, school districts are essentially centralized and linear in their management hierarchy. While district administrators might agree to implement IPM, their commitment to adopt it can be confirmed only by their willingness to communicate what this commitment means to the principals, teachers, students, maintenance, custodial and kitchen staff. Whereas administrators and teachers are normally viewed as education professionals, other staff who would be relied on to conduct cultural, mechanical and sometimes chemical control are not. The custodial staff often are long-term community members who take pride in their jobs. By communicating with them as professionals and giving them control of pest management activities in their schools, they become more committed to the goals of the program.

As mentioned in Chapter Three, I find it interesting that teachers are viewed by administration and the staff as the audience primarily responsible for attracting and maintaining pests. After all, teachers are the only true, long-term human inhabitants of the school buildings. If one wants to find pests, look in the teacher's lounge or in the cupboard of the most beloved kindergarten teacher. I love them, but they are pigs. Of course, students are second only to teachers in their abilities to provide transportation of pests to and their maintenance in the facility (e.g., lunch bags and lockers). Both of these audiences understandably behave in the school somewhat differently than in their primary residences, in that they rely on custodial staff to provide sanitation functions. This frame of reference could be viewed as the primary barrier to communication in this centralized system. However, because of the educational culture inherent in the school community, all audiences are receptive to informational communications that affect the consequences to one's actions—a common classroom phrase.

The following sub-sections describe these stages of the innovation-decision process (figure 5) and demonstrate that, while the message communicated fundamentally remains the same, the media and specific audiences (school administrator, teacher, students/parents and kitchen, custodial and maintenance staff) can change in the process.

• The Knowledge Stage

The knowledge stage begins when individuals in the community become aware of an innovation and how it might work. Typically, awareness occurs through exposure to a mass media technology such as television, radio, or the print media. At this point the sender transmits the message, "Here is a new solution to a problem (old or new)," with the intent of communicating that the innovation (IPM) will meet the community's need. At this stage the primary audience could be the school administration or local change agent.

Figure 5:

THE ACTION TO BE TAKEN:
diffuse IPM

THE INNOVATION/DECISION PROCESS
MODEL ADAPTED FROM ROGERS 1983

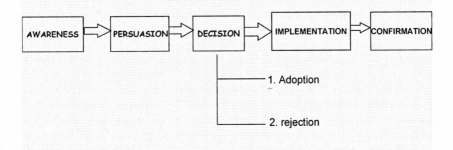

• The Persuasion Stage

The stage at which the adopter unit develops an attitude toward innovation is the persuasion stage. The potential adopter sees the innovation not only as a new idea or practice as defined by Rogers (1983), but also incorporates the idea of risk and uncertainty relative to its application (Downs and Mohr, 1977). If the attitude toward the innovation is positive, it could lead to a change in overt behavior, whereas, if the attitude is negative, it could lead to rejection of the innovation (Lambur, et al., 1985). Interpersonal communication begins to dominate the process at this stage. The audience is presented with the characteristics of the innovation it is being asked to try.

Two specific messages should be sent to audiences: 1) "The presence of pests is a result of their ability to enter your facilities and subsist on the food, water and shelter that you provide for them"; and 2) "By incorporating your knowledge of pests in the performance of your job (sanitation, building maintenance, education, etc.), you can manage pests without increasing your workload." In other much more meaningful words, "Do what you are doing now – just think pests!"

• The Decision Stage

At the decision stage, members of the community decide whether they will adopt the innovation for use in their program. At this point the school district is sending the message, "Yes, you have convinced me/us to try out your new solution". However, a more important exchange is taking place within the communication network of the adopting unit. This is the communication between early adopters (administrators) and later adopters (faculty and staff). Newsletters should be distributed to the schools to reinforce some of the issues addressed in training and presentations. The newsletters contain updates and information about the program and pests in schools. Entertaining facts about insects can be included as well as pest control hints. Testimonies from members of the school community should also be included, as these testimonies prove invaluable. Phrases like, "I've been watching for bugs", "It's just the right thing to do", "It's a no brainer", "I have less work because my teachers aren't complaining about bugs so much" and "We just don't see roaches any more" decide the fate of the adoption.

• The Implementation Stage

The implementation stage is perhaps the most important in the innovation-decision process. Rogers (1995) contends that actually using the idea or practice represents a concrete test of applicability. While Rice and Rogers (1980) believe re-invention may occur at any stage, it is during implementation perhaps more than any other stage that re-invention becomes operational. Implementers include the message, "Yes, you are using this innovation correctly" or "No, but here is how you can make it work properly". At this point, it is critical to avoid information overload. The implementer may recognize, and should accept, that adopters will utilize various coping methods including re-invention. Nurturing may best describe what the change agent must do at this stage.

The change agents need to conduct periodic visits during the next two years. These site visits include inspections for the presence of pests and conditions which could be conducive to pest infestations. Remedial measures should not only be suggested, but observed and critiqued as well. However, visits also are conducted to facilitate communication—both to the change agents from the community and by the change agents to the community regarding pest status/problems, program status/problems. This type of communication extends beyond the actual visits. As with relationships between the extension urban entomologist and the private sector exterminator, these entomologists must make themselves available for questions from the school community — most often from the IPM Coordinator, but occasionally from teachers and staff.

Probably the most important phrase I use during this "hand holding" stage is, "IPM is a process, not a miracle". While the adopters of school IPM have been sold on implementing recommendations for achieving real IPM, they often are uncertain at what pace such actions should occur. For example, achieving the suggested level of sanitation to really prevent pests from being attracted to or allowed to infest the school environment will take training, oversight and time. Further, it is not reasonable to expect maintenance crews to replace all the door sweeps in a school, even in the first year of implementation. We ask school facility managers to address, with appropriate pest monitoring, situations that are most likely to become, or actually are, an infested area. We must remind them that IPM is an ongoing process as with their everyday energy, security and sanitation procedures. This is critical communication and makes your audience more comfortable.

• The Confirmation Stage

The confirmation stage occurs when adopters assure themselves that the decision to adopt was correct. Adopters may decide at any time to discontinue the innovation if it no longer continues to reinforce the adoption. While "location, location, and location" are touted as the three essential aspects of successful restaurants, "feedback, feedback, feedback" might be analogous to confirming the continued use of an innovation. The implementers and community members should gather and exchange information related to the success or failure of the innovation. Pats on the back using mass media or interpersonal communication are necessary.

The USEPA, the National Foundation for IPM education and the IPM Institute of North America have recognized, with award plaques, successful program implementation by school districts that used the Monroe IPM Model. The plaques contain phrases such as, "...for your successful efforts in protecting the children of..." These plaques or letters of congratulation are presented to the supervisor of whomever made the decision to adopt. Further, we often are successful at obtaining news coverage for the award ceremony, A job well done is recognized by newsletters, local newspapers and, when we're lucky, regional or national media.

When we consider both the nature of IPM as an innovation and the findings on adoption practices, two additional policy implications can be mentioned. The first of these relates to the idea that at least two types of information about IPM need to be disseminated. The first type deals with the nature of the innovation itself. This information describes IPM generally and addresses its use and possible benefits. The purpose of this type of information is to spread the idea and influence potential adopters to give IPM a trial. From the perspective of the individual adopter, this type of information is important in getting started on an IPM plan or program. The second type of information regarding IPM deals with the mechanics of individual techniques and their implementation. This information is procedural and lays out not only what needs to be done to initiate a technique, but also what should be done to sustain its use.

From the perspective of developing a dissemination strategy for IPM, both types of information are critically important. Furthermore, since adoptions of an innovation occur at different rates in communities, it is important that both types of information be disseminated simultaneously. In this way, information is available to those who are at the decision stage of the diffusion process and additional information is available to sustain those who have already made adoption decisions. This is accomplished by change agents in two ways: First, ensure that both types of information are continually available — that is, built into the dissemination plan. For instance, promote IPM education to the general public (students and parents) in the context of general awareness of environmental health concerns. Second, be sure to disseminate each type of information. Unless detailed follow-up information is available with this type of innovation, there is a danger that the number of adoptions will begin to approximate the number of discontinuances.

The implication of understanding diffusion as a sub-specialty of communication science is that change agents who implement IPM improve their overall communication skills. As change agents assemble their implementation plan with some emphasis on diffusion, the communication strategy becomes critical. Once these change agents have answered the questions: "What action has to be taken?" "Who is to take it?" and "Do these people have the capacity to do it?" (Starling, 1992, p. 402), the agents, as communicators, then describe the management situation, the audience and preferred medium of communication (Garnett, 1992). A plan involving a conscious observation of diffusion forces communication focus through process. The implementer/change agent necessarily identifies the specific management situation, audience and media by the time the innovation-decision process stage occurs.

Finally, I should note that technological advances that involve the mass media and certain interpersonal media (e.g., interactive television, Internet, cellular telephones) allow more convenient communications between the change agents and the school community — but not necessarily better communication. With the large amount of information one could send out regarding IPM, it becomes critical to avoid information overload.

This concern places the change agent in a position of needing to use more basic and effective forms of face-to-face communication to determine which, and how much, information is needed. In that, in order to converge on a mutual understanding, the change agent eventually must rely on the most basic interpersonal communication, including intonation, facial expression and body language. In my opinion, the most effective communication is usually face to face. Change agents should be prepared to be vulnerable when utilizing this more intimate form of contact. Those who implement IPM should not over-rely on technological devices used for, and sometimes in place of, interpersonal communication. As I tell my students, the best managers will make every attempt to "manage by walking around".

Chapter Six - Building a Better Mousetrap in Indiana - "Do what you are doing now just think pests"

In 1994, several graduate students who had heard one of my lectures on IPM asked me if I could assist them by suggesting a local IPM project with which they could fulfill their program requirements. These students were on a Lilly Community Assistance Fellowship which allowed them to conduct such projects and they were very sharp troops. David Hokanson had just returned from Africa as a Peace Corps Volunteer and Linda Debrewer was one of our environmental chemists. Both knew what IPM was, but more importantly, understood environmental policy and implementation. Having beaten my head against the IPM wall in agriculture and also having tasted the potential that IPM had with public schools in Arizona, I thought trying out a program based on management (particularly communication) would be just the ticket for these students and me. We decided to ask the school district (not, coincidently, where my children were being taught) if we could study conditions there.

The Monroe County Community School Corporation is a school district located in Bloomington, Indiana, home of Indiana University. This large university is a major component of the school community as it pertains to students, teacher training and parental influence of the school board. The school system was made up of 19 schools —14 elementary schools, three middle schools and two high schools. The schools ranged from two to 67 years old and occupancy per structure ranged from 185 to 1,800 students. Total student population of the school corporation was approximately 10,000. We asked the school corporation (a.k.a. district) superintendent for permission to interview school personnel, conduct site assessments and analyze documents related to pest management. Fortunately, the school administration was accustomed to "cooperating" with the university on graduate student projects of all kinds. However, having experienced a costly "sick school syndrome" situation (related to mold in the ventilation system) in 1993, this administration was particularly sensitive to environmental issues involving its schools. The superintendent readily agreed to cooperate and assigned his Planning Director, John Carter, to assist us. The second major step in this program's development was to include entomologists from Purdue University — after an in-depth economic and pest management audit by the grad students.

John seemed to be pretty interested in this IPM stuff, and he arranged for Dave and Linda to have access to all the information the school district had dealing with pest management and even instructed the school faculty and staff to cooperate. Dave and Linda found that 83% of the schools had pest populations which were in need of treatment; there were reports of roaches crawling out of desks. According to pest control contractors, the predominant pests were roaches and rodents. Survey responses from the school occupants indicated that Yellow Jackets and bees were the pests most frequently reported, followed by roaches and ants.

The district used one nationally known pest control firm and two local pest control firms to manage pests. Although the district moved away from in-house pesticide application, custodians did do some spraying. The pest control operators conducted routine, monthly spraying of all buildings, generally without regard to pest presence or biology. The effectiveness of the exterminator was questioned only when problems or complaints arose. The exterminators visited schools after hours and at the end of the school week to avoid potential pesticide complaints. Records showed that these exterminators did not always use pesticides that presented minimum health and environmental exposure risks (Debrewer & Hokanson, 1995). Some pesticides, such as weed killer and wasp spray, were even sent to individual schools by extended services. In fact, schools were sometimes allowed to buy their own pesticides, as was the case schools that had large athletic fields. Supplying products to schools and purchasing pesticides for schools was done informally, not subject to any formal guidelines.

It appeared that spending for pest management did not constitute much of the district's overall budget, but it did comprise a considerable amount of the total maintenance budget. Total costs associated with pests included payment to contractors, wages for custodial personnel (including only time devoted to pest control), costs of pest control equipment and repair costs for damage caused by pests.

The largest portion of pest control costs was associated with payment to contractors and school personnel involved in pest control-related activities (such as pest removal, cleaning, plugging holes, etc.). The amount spent on contractors was approximately $32,000 annually for pest control (including termite control). It was not clear whether the district formally compared increased costs to improvement in pest control when changing contractors. There appeared to be a large jump in contractor payments that occurred when the contractor was changed. There was little quality control for pest management, and the school faculty and staff were not aware of the pest control applicator's responsibilities, which made it very difficult for the schools to evaluate the efficiency of pest control measures in place. As a result, contractor performance was measured by the school in terms of anecdotal evidence (Hokanson & Debrewer, 1996).

Based on the assessments, we recommended that the school district consider implementing a pilot program to determine if IPM was the right approach for the school system. The administration agreed, with the standard "Okay, as long as it doesn't cost us anything". Timing couldn't have been better. I contacted my old friend Ralph Wright with the Office of Pesticide Programs at USEPA headquarters and "put the arm on him" — we needed money and I was willing to whine a lot. Ralph informed me about a relatively new program – Pesticide Environmental Stewardship Program (PESP) which was set up for just the kind of IPM program we were interested in. So I called the PESP partnership guy, who as it happened was accepting grant proposals that very week. Turns out it was an old cotton IPM aquaintance from Texas – Mike Wallace – now with the National Foundation for IPM Education. Both Mike and Ralph advised me to hurry and make sure the proposal would actually accomplish something, rather than just studying it. My students had already conducted the study. We were ready to really sink our teeth into demonstrating school IPM.

Giving Birth – Program Formulation

The Partners

I figured once the students' evaluation of Monroe County Community School Corporation's pest management was really working well and the school administration was demonstrating commitment our next step would be to involve Indiana's land grant Cooperative Extension institution — Purdue. The IPM and Urban Entomology specialists needed to be involved so they could provide technical input and program implementation strategies and determine possible implications of the program.

Purdue had a reputation for assembling some of the best materials in the country for agricultural IPM, and I was really looking forward to working with them. I have mentioned how much Extension feels it owns IPM, so I viewed it as a real professional courtesy when four of their entomologists agreed to meet with me about this project. The lead guy on urban pest management at Purdue is Gary Bennett. He brought several of his associates he wanted to be directly involved: Tim Gibb, Bobby Corrigan and Fred Whitford, who is the Pesticide Applicator Training specialist. I laid out the situation in Bloomington and suggested that we use USEPA, Office of Pesticide Programs, Pesticide Environmental Stewardship Program grant money to develop a pilot program. It turns out that they were very interested in school IPM. Fred even had a school district with a possible pesticide-related death of a student, and there was some serious political pressure on Purdue to begin to address pesticides in schools. However, while they had conducted a survey on the subject, no one had attempted to develop or implement an actual school IPM program.

It looked like we had ourselves an implementation team. Tim is really a turf and ornamental management specialist; however he's also well-trained in urban pest management. Since he's Canadian we all had to talk very slowly when explaining American pests to Tim. Fortunately, he was on the school board up in Tippecanoe County and had some political insight into how those elected officials made decisions. Tim would become the director of a USEPA-funded school IPM center at Purdue, which would assist in implementing IPM in the Midwest. Bobby was just finishing his Ph.D., working on rodent pest management, and had the down and dirty experience of an inner city exterminator. Further, he had taken it on himself to become educated as a building sanitarian, and was already consulting with some major food processing companies who could not have pests in their products nor pesticide residue on those products. Bobby had assisted Gary with writing the book on pest control operations. He would soon graduate and start the RMC Pest Management consulting firm we worked with for the next seven years. Fred was a former regulator with the Louisiana State Lead Agency and had lots of experience with structural pest control. He is an incredible resource on pesticides and their effects on humans and the environment. Fred is one of the most entertaining speakers you will ever hear — lots of "down home" humor and an in-your-face style of communication. He loves teaching and always looks like he has been crawling around in something. John Carter just plain cared about his school district, knew there had to be a better way to control pests (he had stories of kids consistently missing school the day after pesticides were sprayed in classrooms) and seemed to get a kick out of watching us bug guys do our thing. John knows how schools are run (in the hallways and boardrooms) and how to find out what is really going on with people and funding. Besides, we needed someone who actually wore a tie every day. Dave and Linda were very excited about seeing if their evaluation could really make a difference, and I was back in the IPM business. So we went to work outlining an implementation plan (based on the evaluation already conducted by Dave and Linda) with the following proposed strategies:

How we did it.

- Chose three schools to represent the district as pilot schools
- Monitored each school for common pests
- Assessed each school for conditions conducive to pest entry and infestation
- Agreed on management strategies for any infestations
- Recommended remediation strategies for any conducive condition
- Trained the pilot school staff to recognize pests, pest infestations and conducive conditions
- Developed and disseminated a "pest press" newsletter for faculty and staff
- Evaluated the success of the pilot program and communicated the results to the appropriate people

The schools we picked were ones with the worst pest problems. Fairview Elementary was built in the 1920s; it had mice, Pavement Ants, Yellow Jacket paper wasps and German and Oriental Cockroaches as chronic pests. It is interesting how we usually hear that old schools are the worst for pests (as if the implementation of management strategies like good sanitation and exclusion cannot work in older buildings). However, we found that Fairview was in pretty good shape and would turn out to be one of our model schools. Binford Elementary was built in the '50s and was in rough shape. One of its worst problems was that it had utility tunnels, which pests love. Binford had the same chronic pests as Fairview and also a fierce fruit fly problem. Bloomington South High School had all the pests we found at the other schools – just more of them. In particular, mice plagued the school. They entered under doors that should have been fitted better or had better doorsweeps. Roaches owned the kitchens.

The conditions in these three schools that attracted and maintained pests were not too bad compared to those of many other schools in the United States. We found that sanitation was good to superior, based on Bobby's evaluation. Most of the pest problems were related to food storage and classroom clutter. Unfortunately, teachers without budgets for classroom materials become pack rats and seldom throw anything away. Further, they know the best reward for themselves and their students is the snack. Nice folks, but when it comes to the cause and effect relationship with pests, they couldn't add two and two. The kitchens and custodial closets were a bit of a problem. Drains were dirty and mops were stored improperly — they needed to be free of debris, with the mop head up off the floor and handle down. Interestingly, Fairview's sanitation was the best. The reason for this was that the head custodian was a "white tornado" and made damn' sure her staff kept up — a lesson we did not forget. With the best intentions, all the schools recycled soda cans in boxes in the cafeterias. Syrup from the cans leaked through the boxes on to the floor and attracted ants and fruit flies. Teachers' lounges were dirty. The teachers stored food in open containers and did not clean up after themselves. Of course these lounges contained old refrigerators, couches and vending machines for lonely, cold and hungry cockroaches, mice and spiders that also were looking for some place to fall in love and start a family. Trash management was good, but the trash bags were cheap and broke apart when tossed into the dumpsters, so the dumpsters themselves were filthy. They and the areas around them became a friendly place for houseflies, their little maggot babies, Yellow Jackets, rats, mice and crows. This is a real problem when the trash is stored right outside the kitchen door, as it is with most schools. The pests would enter the kitchen, particularly when the doors were propped open in warm weather. Yellow Jacket wasps were a chronic problem in all the trash containers placed on school grounds for the students to use. They had become a very convenient stop for foraging insects. All in all, the schools looked clean, but more so to the human eye than from the pest point of view.

Believe it or not, the fixes for pest problems in these three schools were pretty easy. We needed to concentrate on sanitation and exclusion practices and integrate a very temporary chemical control practice. John procured better trash bags, better trash cans for student use, better doorsweeps and less pest-conducive shelving for the kitchens. He required delivery of cleaner and better-maintained dumpsters from his trash hauler, and mandated in-service sanitation training for the custodial staff at each school. Finally, he allowed Linda and Dave to distribute issues of the Pest Press they had written to the pilot school faculty and staff, and communicated a policy for clutter control as well as the prohibition of any pesticide application other than by the new IPM coordinator. This is what I mean by having a partner in the school district for successful IPM implementation.

We decided early in this program that a former maintenance supervisor, Jerry Jochim, would obtain his Pest Control Operator's (PCO) license and be further trained by Bobby Corrigan and me in the people management and technical pest management required for real IPM. The Pesticide Environmental Stewardship Program funding allowed for Jerry's special training and transition into the in-house IPM coordinator position. As mentioned in chapter four, Jerry became our star pupil and a major contributor to the national implementation of IPM in schools. However, one of our first practical field experiences with him yielded a procedure that appeared to be "ass backwards" to those we had been teaching him.

Because the cockroach population was so high in several of our schools, Bobby taught Jerry how to apply cockroach bait properly. If applied where the roach forages and resides (based on species and life stage), this pesticide bait can be used in tiny amounts more effectively than pesticides an uneducated exterminator might use and certainly more effectively than using a liquid or aerosol. Those methods not only can be dangerous but also can actually disperse roaches to other parts of the structure. Based on our monitoring traps, Bobby and Jerry baited the schools...and, as you will read, it would virtually be for the last time.

By developing the IPM coordinator position, the program was able to eliminate a number of serious communication barriers. In the pre-program assessment, it had been established that outside contractors (several nationally known firms) did not adequately communicate with the school community. This actually was understandable since the exterminators held a different frame of reference. To them, pest management meant controlling pests rather than managing people. They spent little time in the schools and simply were not members of the school community. We strongly believed that monitoring and education were fundamental to IPM and could be more effectively accomplished by a member of the school community. This really upset the exterminators working with the school district. Although we offered to let them join us on a "retainer" basis, they refused and swore John would beg to have them back within the year.

Our training session with the custodians went great. It was a very laid-back intro to the causes of pest problems and what IPM truly is. We agreed before training that the best message to send this audience was, "you can do what you're doing now, just think pests!"— but with the critical understanding that we were dealing with professionals in the school community. Fred demonstrated how the custodians distributed pesticides on their hands and clothes when they improperly used pesticides; Tim talked about how IPM fit into their school situation; and Bobby enhanced their appetites with a discussion on how mice pee on the surface of desks and whatever might be inside the desks and cupboards (silverware and open food included). We were talking sanitation and exclusion from the pests' point of view. It was my job to convince them that they could incorporate pest prevention, pest monitoring and pest control into their existing jobs of security, sanitation and building repair. It seemed to strike a chord when I mentioned, "teachers are pigs" (sorry, Aunt Pauline). At that point, the custodians figured we knew what we were talking about.

Finally, I began a campaign to develop program recognition with some news reporters in Indiana, and with the Indiana Department of Environmental Management. This strategy was to confirm to the school system that it had made the right decision to adopt. I began wondering if I had made the right decision to develop this team and move so aggressively, because I really didn't know if this thing would work as well as I hoped. None of us did. That's why they call it risk taking.

Results

With these strategies and incredibly good partnership, the pilot schools demonstrated an almost immediate decrease in pest complaints and a drastic decrease in pesticide use. After only six months into the pilot program, the Monroe County Community School Corporation decided to implement IPM in all of its schools (figure 6 on the Appendix cover page). In the first year of the district-wide program, inspections confirmed that some of the general sanitation technologies discussed in training had been adopted by custodial staff. Many of the technologies, however, were already in use prior to the program and therefore showed no change. Classroom sanitation technologies also were being used at a high pre-existing rate, so little new adoption occurred in this area — "just think pests!" However, custodial staff did recognize that teachers were making efforts to reduce clutter in their classrooms. Repair and exclusion technologies such as installing proper doorsweeps were slowly implemented. One reason for this was the timing and procedure for repair requests. Although Extended Services agreed to expedite requests from program schools, caulking and some repairs could not be performed during the winter months, and thus were delayed until spring and summer.

Policies were developed and implemented for the use of pesticides. These included the requirement that any presence of pests was to be reported to the IPM coordinator, and insecticide applications were to be made only by Jerry. He also eliminated the use of all scheduled treatments, aerosols and broadcast liquid applications within the facilities. Any pesticide treatments were to be applied only in response to monitoring data. Reports and confirmation of pest infestations were reduced to less than one per school. Pre-program applications of insecticides for the school district (1992-1994) averaged 10 per school or approximately 180 per year for the district. Two-year, post-pilot program data revealed total applications of insecticides in the 18 schools of the district were 15. By the most conservative calculation of using the pre-program yearly total compared to the IPM program two-year total, there appeared to be a 92% reduction in insecticide use accompanied by a 90% reduction in pest complaints.

The Bottom Line – Cost and Benefits to the School District incurred from its implementation of IPM

Many school districts have claimed that IPM has saved them thousands of dollars per year; however, no analyses have yet been published. It is recognized by those who implemented IPM that these claims tend to be biased, as they do not include variables such as custodial time, reduced health risks, or decreased maintenance costs. Therefore, to assess the accuracy of these claims, a detailed benefit cost analysis of the Monroe County Community School Corporation was prepared in 1999 and 2003.

Estimating the costs of the program was perhaps the most difficult analysis of this case. This study was conducted in 1999 by another graduate fellow, Terry Lumish. Her cost/benefit analysis of the Monroe County Community School Corporation's experience with IPM determined that the benefits of IPM savings to the district amounted to approximately $9,000 over the course of six years. This included the addition of the salaried IPM coordinator position. Her model accounted for both direct and indirect costs. Examples of costs for the IPM strategy included the following:

- moving waste receptacles away from the facility;
- installing physical barriers such as air curtains;
- improving structural maintenance (leaky pipes and torn screens, for example);
- IPM training requiring time away from work;
- Internet use;
- re-landscaping next to buildings;

- monitoring and bait stations;
- pesticides, when necessary;
- protective equipment for custodians;
- sealants and other maintenance supplies;
- containers and other materials for pest exclusion;
- newsletters and other literature for staff training and use; and
- health insurance premiums.

Other factors considered in this analysis included the number of children affected, the number of facilities within the school district, the size of facilities, square footage and number of classrooms, additional personnel requirements and the percentage of time employees dedicated to IPM. Some costs were one-time expenditures for implementation, while others were ongoing so as to achieve and sustain the successful IPM program.

Through a step-wise process, the model accounted for the time, equipment, chemicals and education for a number of stakeholders within the school system. These included its custodians, maintenance employees, administration, kitchen staff, pest industry contractors, faculty members, students and parents. The costs and benefits incurred by each party were determined for both the traditional (exterminator) and IPM options. Many required costs already were included in the school corporation's annual budget. Some of these were required or recommended by the health department or other public officials to promote safe, secure facilities. It was determined that the system's insurance company would neither increase liability for doing more pest management work in-house, nor would it reduce rates if the school corporation changed its pest management policies.

Terry's conclusion was, "Comparing the traditional pest management benefit value to the IPM costs for the same time period resulted in a benefit-cost ratio of 1:1. Because IPM is more cost-effective than the established pest control program (that is, it provides the MCCSC with greater bang for its buck), it is in the district's interest to adopt this alternative program. IPM is less expensive, while offering the benefits detailed above." The bottom line in this analysis was that IPM is cost-effective for the short and long terms in well-managed schools, but demonstrates a greater long-term benefit (rather than short) for schools that are not well managed (Lumish and Lame, 1999). In 2003 another cost/benefit analysis was conducted by Kristi Kubista which found even more significant benefits accrued to the Bloomington school district after it adopted IPM. This substantiated our previous finding that IPM is more cost-effective in schools that demonstrate an overall good level of facilities management in all areas.

NUMBERS!

Kristi found that IPM is cost effective in schools where 10 percent of the maintenance staff's time is spent dealing with pest-related activities (i.e., pesticide application, repairing damaged materials, or talking with teachers and students) and one percent of the equipment budget is spent fixing pest-related damage that occurred before IPM was implemented. In school districts where pests don't exist, IPM appears less cost effective than more traditional approaches since the maintenance costs are so low, and custodial, teacher and kitchen staff monitoring costs must be considered when IPM is implemented.

This is not to say that school districts that experience few or no pests cannot experience a catastrophic pesticide misuse or dangerous pest incident, which could result from a negligent pest control program. We were not able to assess these factors. Further, these results ignore other major unquantifiable variables, such as the benefits of decreased absenteeism, better safety controls, educational benefits for teachers, students and parents, easily accessible record keeping, increased sanitation and energy conservation standards and the long-term health benefits associated with decreased pesticide exposures. As part of the cost/benefit analysis, regressions were run on absentee rates and the existence of IPM. Although the relationship is occluded by many other variables that affect the school district, IPM does show signs that it decreases absentee rates. If these variables were to be quantified, IPM would most likely demonstrate significant cost/benefit performance for all school districts.

This cost/benefit analysis can easily be transferred to other school districts that operate in a manner similar to Bloomington in Monroe County, Indiana. One employee, or IPM coordinator, spends 50 percent of his/her time on IPM-related activities. Another, the administrator of custodial maintenance, spends 10 percent of his time on IPM activities. Custodial and kitchen staff spend 12.3 hours per year on IPM activities, along with one hour of training a year, taught by the IPM coordinator. This cost/benefit analysis, depending on whether completed for larger or smaller schools, may have different numerical results, but the positive or negative signs remain the same. Numerical values were calculated from ratios that in most situations will be similar for all school districts. The variables used in the cost/benefit analysis can be divided into two categories: the positives and negatives of IPM.

The positive variables included in this analysis were absentee rates for students and staff, awards and recognition, long-term health benefits, more effective pest management, increased safety, direct asthma savings, indirect asthma savings, indoor/outdoor total pesticide-related expenditure savings, student and teacher education, herbicide savings, accountable record keeping and grant money.

The negative variables included grant writing costs, implementer salaries, dissemination and outreach, travel costs, implementing supplies, educational IPM letters, parent notification letters, parent/board meetings, the administrator's time, the IPM Coordinator's time, staff/faculty educational IPM newsletters, teacher monitoring time, kitchen staff maintenance and observation time, custodial maintenance and observation time, training of kitchen staff, training of custodians, pesticide and program maintenance costs and start-up costs of the program.

Unfortunately, not enough research has been completed to quantify many of the benefits, although all of the costs have numerical values. This of course, allows IPM opponents to portray IPM as less cost-effective. If numerical values could replace these unquantified variables, using economics to convince school districts to implement IPM would be even more effective.

Communication and Recognition

In terms of communication, the program was exceptional. One-on-one communication was very effective with the custodial staff. We did make one major mistake by not including the kitchen staff during our first year of the program, and it is always a bad mistake to ignore the cooks. It really did delay some of our food storage and management issues in the pantries. Newsletters were informative, but personal contact seemed to be preferred. The custodial staff seemed comfortable asking questions and taking advice from Jerry and the other team members regarding pest management. The school staff were quite receptive to the program. They originally thought that the integrated approach to pest management would add to their workload. During the program, that perception changed. Anecdotally, they were proud that pests and pesticides had been reduced in their schools. The positive consequences of their actions confirmed their adoption of the program (Hokanson and Debrewer, 1996). The message, "Tools you will be learning and using to prevent pests in your schools will also work for your home" really did stimulate principals, faculty and staff to take an interest in our visits and newsletters.

Awards and recognition definitely did seal the deal with the school community. Jerry now has an annual custodial appreciation day for the district staff. The school system has received awards from Indiana's governor for pollution prevention and from the National Foundation for IPM Education and the USEPA for protecting the children of Indiana. No fewer than 12 articles appeared in local, state and national periodicals, and the school system is prominently featured in the USEPA, Office of Pesticide Program's brochure on IPM in schools. Show me a school board or superintendent anywhere in the country that wouldn't adopt a program for these warm and fuzzy political gifts. However, in the case of Monroe County and as you will read, in numerous other school communities, the adoption of real IPM was because "it is the right thing to do". And, by including John and Jerry implementing the Monroe IPM Model in other school corporations, as well as day-care centers in Indiana and other locations around the country, they had become IPM Evangelists — they could never go back.

Chapter Seven — Sneaking Back into Arizona — Testing the IPM Model

I needed a school district that was similar to Monroe County but in a new location with different change agents in order to test the model we had built in Bloomington. However, I did not have the time or money to build relationships from the ground up. John Carter at Monroe County agreed to propose a Pesticide Environmental Stewardship Program grant to the USEPA to show that we could transfer our success in Bloomington to other states. Since I had contacts in Arizona and Alabama I figured we could get things going pretty quickly in those locations. I had no certainty it would work, but knew we had real believers in both states.

As part of the grant (I did mention that this money was about as much as the cost of a new SUV), we had two major objectives:

1) To demonstrate the IPM innovation (using the Monroe IPM Model) to public educations communities in states currently practicing IPM in schools by coordinating/implementing a successful pilot program in representative schools.

2) To educate entities (change agents) involved with implementing IPM (State Lead Agencies, Extension, Pest Control Operators, and Public Health, others...) about program initiation, implementation and evaluation of IPM in the public school environment (Lame, 1999).

These objectives were to be accomplished through:

EDUCATION:
- Training change agents in both states to assess and implement public school IPM programs.
- Training staff at schools in Arizona and Alabama to incorporate IPM in their existing operational activities (sanitation, maintenance, food service, health and education).
- Training those who provide pest control technology (pest monitoring and pesticide application) with state-of-the-art methods and tools for use in child-sensitive facilities.

DEMONSTRATION:
- Demonstrating IPM program planning, implementation and assessment to State Lead Agencies and school districts in Arizona and Alabama through the successful implementation of an IPM pilot program in representative school districts (Lame, 1999).

Sneaking Back into Arizona

I have a love/hate relationship with Arizona. I love the state— its weather, ecosystems and history (natural and social), but I HATE what has happened to it. An economy based on uncontrolled growth has raped the southwestern beauty and charm I grew up with in the 1960s. In saying this I realize the Arizona Department of Tourism will not feel compelled to display this book in its lobby. As a youngster I could dream of no more an exciting place to grow up, and as a middle-aged man I resent what that place has become.

Moving to the outskirts of Tempe from Hudson, Ohio, in 1966 allowed me to experience many of the exotic fantasies of a 13-year-old "nature boy". The desert (a 10-minute bike ride through the barrio of Guadalupe) was a place of wonder and excitement. My ride to the desert was a movie set from my youth —Yaqui Indians, Mexican immigrants and the snakes, lizards and cacti with which my adventure heroes co-existed. To me, venomous animals were very exciting, be they rattlesnakes, scorpions, Gila Monsters, or tarantulas. I caught them all and took them home where I kept them in my refrigerator until I could present them to Dr. Stahnke's lab at Arizona State University. Stahnke conducted research on venomous animals and paid me 25 cents per animal. Dangerous animals and good money! Actually, the really dangerous animal was my mother who had some weird problem with live rattlesnakes in her fridge (my wife seems to have inherited this problem, as I still occasionally store collected insects for identification).

Kyrene School was a light-green school house south of Tempe back when I used to ride my bike past it. Now it is a school district for the children of "boomers" that moved to the "southeast valley" in the '70s, '80s, and '90s. Most of the desert and agricultural habitat of my glorious venomous friends is now houses and strip malls, but many of these animals (particularly the arthropods) are very adaptive, and they have moved in with the boomers. They have become pests. Not only that, but civilization has provided a more diverse habitat that also supports various ant and roach species, lice, houseflies, black widow spiders, filth flies, Indian House Crickets and other pests common to our human species. The 26 Kyrene schools had all of these pests and were spraying the hell out of them to no avail.

The Players

Change Agents

Back to IPM. I knew Extension entomologists at the University of Arizona and I watched Kyrene grow up. I was pretty sure I knew the pest problems involved. Further, I figured I could talk my old IPM buddy, Mike Lindsey, into becoming an on-site coordinator for the project. Besides our work in cotton, Mike worked with me and Maude on one of the first school IPM programs in 1992 in Paradise Valley. The administration there was pretty ugly and eventually went for the low bid after Mike had showed them how to do things right. We were both aching to show what IPM really could do in the right school district.

Paul Baker was a former faculty colleague of mine from Tucson and a damn' fine termite man. He readily jumped at the chance to try IPM in the schools. Fortunately for all of us, the department had just hired Dawn Gouge as their new Urban Entomologist. We all agreed that Dawn would spearhead the Extension effort from the university.

The State Lead Agency in Arizona is the Structural Pest Control Board. It was pretty good ol' boy when it comes to IPM. Carl Martin was a recent hire, was gung ho about IPM, and didn't really care that his agency wasn't involved. He brought his people into our program. Just to make sure they kept their end of the deal, I talked Mary Grisier from USEPA, Office of Pesticide Programs Region 9 out of San Francisco, into assisting our team. Mary's office reviews the State Lead Agencies in her region for compliance with FIFRA. Mary was able to help us all cope with the federal bureaucracy — no small task. Being a former regulatory official and knowing how the pest control industry in Arizona worked, I figured Carl's administration would drag its feet on this project. So I drew up a Memorandum of Understanding that required the change agents to provide:

- Onsite coordination and communication with regard to information dissemination in the program area.
- Data gathering/sharing in the context of existing or ongoing economic and pest surveys dealing with pest management in schools.
- Willingness to coordinate activities with other states (dependent on travel funding).
- Tailoring this program to their state, albeit within the confines of the Monroe IPM Model parameters.
- Bi-weekly communication with an IPM implementation team member.
- Attendance and participation in at least one training session and one on-site inspection (MOU, Appendix D)

In return, I offered to provide training free of charge and create a public relations climate that would publicize their willingness to protect the children of Arizona.

The School District

Kyrene School District consists of 26 schools serving a mostly middle and upper middle class community. From my point of view, it is a well-managed suburban school district. Approaching the district administration was too easy. I called Stan Peterson, the facilities manager, told him what I proposed and asked for an appointment. Stan is one laid-back guy, a real pro and a risk taker. I described the Monroe IPM model to him and asked if we could try it at Kyrene. I assured him it wouldn't cost him anything to try it and I would bring the best team in the country in to make it work (some people will believe anything). I gave him John Carter's phone number and asked him to call John to find out what a peer thought about the program. I followed up with a formal letter requesting a partnership. We were on.

We began our project in April, 2000. The first thing I did was produce our Memorandum of Understanding stating that we would provide economic and technical assessments and train the Pest Control contractor and custodial staff of the three pilot schools cost-free. It also said that upon successful completion of the pilot program we would generate press coverage IF the school district desired it. The MOU required the school district to provide:

- Access to previous records related to pest management and pesticide use.
- Access to three schools for inspection and pest management.
- Access to personnel in those schools (mostly staff vs. teachers) for training and determining pest problems.
- Assurance that current Pest Control technicians would be prohibited from treating any of the pilot schools without justification and/or communication with our team (though we welcomed their participation in our training).
- Allow distribution of IPM materials (newsletters) to teachers, administration and staff.
- Agree to visits by school administrators from other states.
- Become a Pesticide Environmental Stewardship Program partner upon successful completion of the pilot program (MOU, Appendix D).

The Pest Control Operators

By now, you will not be surprised at what we found. However, the industry was very sensitive to our criticisms and the fact that Monroe County school district "internalized" pest management. We were trying to listen to the pest control industry's message ("modern pest control firms really aren't exterminators anymore") — and give them the benefit of the doubt. Nice try. What we found confirmed our earlier beliefs about what was going on in schools: the pest control contract could be a license to steal. The exterminators did show up at our first meeting, and when we outlined what we intended to investigate and demonstrate, we never saw them again.

When we originally asked Stan how Kyrene contractors were managing pests, he told us that they "cleaned out" the buildings every summer and then sprayed designated areas every month. The contract was for approximately $400 per school per year — a low bid. Upon hearing this we knew IPM was not being practiced in this school district. "Clean out" meant that the exterminator applied chemical pesticides throughout every school right before the children came back at the end of the summer. There was no indication that pests were being found throughout the school or that there were any fewer pests after the clean out. Why? Because no one was monitoring for pests anywhere in the school district.

I guess because there was no monitoring, exterminators every month would simply spray in traditional areas (kitchen, pantry, bathrooms and administrative offices) and wherever else the custodian told them (if they ever spoke to them) or where teachers, cooks or parents (in the case of "booster" concession rooms) might complain about. If exterminators were told to spray anywhere beyond the low bid contract specifications, they charged more — about $300 per school per year on average. It was interesting to review their invoices. Very much like MCCSC, pre-IPM, the exterminators always found something to charge for, every month. So each school had either 10 extra charges or 12 extra charges, depending on whether it was on a 10- or 12-month schedule. No wonder these guys saw no need to work within our MOU, which required them to document and communicate the justification prior to any pesticide application. There were no written reports about pest-conducive conditions or any confirmation by custodians of any attempt by exterminators to educate school personnel. It was the "wham, bam, thank you, ma'am" method of pest control: spray and run.

Some exterminators I know try to defend this method by saying that school districts that accept low bid contracts get what they pay for. Horse-pucky! It is one thing to take money knowing you won't be able to adequately control pests. It is quite another to demand more money to spray more for no documented reason and possibly create a hazardous situation for children via pesticide exposure and uncontrolled harmful pests. The icing on the cake was that under Arizona law the schools had to post notices of pesticide applications on school grounds for each application. We estimated that such postings cost approximately $300 in staff time (paperwork and physical posting) each year for each school. The bottom line was that exterminators were charging the school district $1,000 per school per year to control pests. Control pests? Not even close.

Pests and Conducive Conditions (diagnosis and education)

Technical assessments are one of the big rewards I get for conducting this type of program. Why? Because I get to be an entomologist. In each pilot school Bobby Corrigan and I worked with our implementation team to technically access the school for what kind of pests it had, the severity of any pest infestation and conditions conducive to causing or maintaining pest infestations (Bennett, 2003). This is critical to our model in terms of diagnosing the pest situation and training our team. It's diagnosis and education.

First, we conducted a history of the pest conditions at the school by reviewing invoices from the Pest Control contractor and interviewing administrators, grounds, custodial, kitchen and maintenance staff. Sometimes we talked to school nurses if they could be found. Most of our answers were at the level of "large red ant versus small black ant", "fly versus beetle or roach" and "mouse versus rat". "Eliciting a physical description of the pest is a communication skill (some would call it an art) much like when a doctor figures out what might be ailing you by asking you where it hurts, and what the hurt feels like. Most folks didn't think they could help us because they don't know "bug talk" or they were too scared or disgusted when they saw the pest. That is exactly what we were counting on — people remember a lot more when they are impressed. It is just a matter of asking the right question. Communication!

We all have different styles, and as the staff guided us through their school, we tried to educate them in our quaint, bug-like ways. Folks love Bobby. He is an Irish New Yorker who encourages his target audience to make fun of his hard-core neighborhood accent and appearance. Some say Bobby even looks like a rat (sorry, bud). Of course, his story of crawling around the sewers of New York looking for and being attacked by rats transforms his appearance. He asks questions such as, "Is the poop you found behind the pantry shelves tapered on the ends or square?" This has something to do with mammals having sphincter muscles and insects not having them. On the other hand, I play the role of squeamish professor. I ask them, "How big are the maggots in your floor drain?" Who ever gets asked that? Bobby will crawl up through the ceiling tiles and I might crawl (and get stuck) under the dishwasher. Mike talks to the dead mice left in bait stations by exterminators who forgot to check them. Jerry will "aw shucks" them with a mouth full of Hoosier 'possum, but very clearly demonstrate he understands how they feel about cleaning floor drains. As she "teases out" a Black Widow spider, Dawn speaks in an English dialect so thick that no one knows whether she is swearing or praying to the gods of lost bugs. The people we interview usually haven't met folks like us before, and they know we are having fun doing our jobs. We even wear costumes — kneepads, bump caps and tool belts with strange tools. Clowns, we might be. WE ARE THE ENTERTAINMENT, and they enjoy participating in the show. Communication!

We normally ask our guides to lead us to the Pest Vulnerable Areas before we check out more general school areas —kitchens, pantries, custodial closets, concession rooms and biology classrooms (dead animals and live animals with their food). Places you might not think would qualify as Pest Vulnerable Areas are teachers' lounges, which usually are pig sties, and vending machine areas, which always produce neat critters. After the Pest Vulnerable Areas, we usually look at places where everyone thinks bugs live, like bathrooms (very little food and harborage) in terms of drains, water leaks and examples of poor sealing (escutcheon plates, etc.). I can't tell you how much fun it is to watch someone like Bobby "work" an area. He'll walk into a kitchen and begin sniffing! Yes, roaches and other pests have distinct odors. Then, to the chagrin and amazement of the custodial staff, he'll often find filthy areas in an otherwise clean looking room — areas that faculty or staff thought were too hidden or difficult to clean. "Where the bugs are" (isn't that a song by Connie Stevens?) will be where people don't clean.

We use our senses to identify pests and infestations, smelling roaches, mouse urine and even the telltale odor of certain ants when crushed. Visual cues are as important as actually hearing termites or wood boring beetles. Sensory inspection works indoors or outdoors. Brought up as an urban entomologist, Bobby views the building as an ecosystem in which he can observe the interaction between living and non-living things (Odum, 1971), just as I would a cotton farm. What allowed the pests to exist and reproduce in this area? What did they eat, drink and take shelter in? Where can they hide and how do they move from room to room? (Corrigan, 2001) With our powers of observation and deduction we got to play scientists!

After looking at the inside of the building we walked the outside perimeter to observe possible points of entry, harborage and attraction. Are the doors and windows sealed properly? Does the landscape (groundcover, trees, shrubs and mulch) provide harborage? Do open trashcans attract Yellow Jacket wasps? Are exterior lights attracting nocturnal insects and are those lights located above doors that are opened often or not sealed correctly? All of our observations were recorded. We developed a strategy for each pest and suggested remediation for each conducive condition.

At Kyrene we found a lot of pests. We identified three types of roaches: American Cockroaches (associated with sewers and irrigation) used the "slab" recreational area outside the cafeteria and became frequent invaders of the building. German Cockroaches were brought into the building in food containers and infested the darker, warmer, damper parts of the school (kitchen, pantry, vending machines!). The Turkistan Roach, relatively new to the Southwest, is a strong night flyer, attracted to outside lights. It often flew in through open kitchen doors. Two species of ants that presented minor problems outdoors were the Southern Fire Ant and Harvester Ants. Really not much of a problem unless you were sitting on or near the mound. However, the Odorous House Ant did invade the building, foraging on food stuff not properly cleaned up — spilled soda, pieces of candy, crumbs, etc. Africanized Bees (a.k.a. Killer Bees) were serious but rare, problems. Of serious concern and not so rare were feral cats that some teachers and students encouraged to live under portable classrooms. Some Norway Rats and House Mice were reported. Pigeons nested in the pavilion above the picnic tables. Indian House Crickets were common, fed on the same stuff as the German Roaches and provided a food source for an uncommonly high number of scorpions. Scorpion stings had been reported, and we found scorpions even in florescent light covers in hallways. Black Widow Spiders abounded, as they are a very common spider associated with structures in the Southwest. Filth flies and fruit flies were common in kitchen areas that didn't properly rotate fruit, improperly disposed of soda cans or failed to keep drains clean. That was the extent of our diagnosis.

The schools looked clean, but only at the human level, not at the pest level. Many conditions allowed entry, feeding, reproduction and shelter. Our biggest problem was getting the school inhabitants — administration, teachers, staff and students — to understand the cause and effect relationship between pests and conducive conditions. This was our education component.

How the Program Progressed

Communication is the core of our program. Once we knew the pest, pesticide and economic situation, we could work to influence the behavior of the school community so they could embrace IPM painlessly. First, we had to substantiate linkage between pests and what the school inhabitants were doing to cause or maintain those pests. We conducted two education and training programs for:

1) Pilot school maintenance, custodial and food service staff .A half-day sit-down and walk-through workshop dealt with pests that were found in the three pilot schools, and principles of IPM pertinent to sanitation and exclusion.

2) Three University of Arizona Extension IPM specialists who got hands-on training from Bobby (on IPM particular to the school pests and the specific pilot school environment) and from me on how to implement this model. Dawn developed and distributed two school newsletters and a statewide manual/newsletter, "Critters Corner".

I communicated bi-weekly with the state program partners — with the exception of the State Lead Agency. Most communication with

Mike was limited to the technical aspects of IPM, and with Dawn and Stan Peterson to program coordination. Although this communication is critical, it became apparent that the state program partners were not communicating for optimal program performance. "Unfortunately, the State Lead Agency's leadership has been in a period of transition. Thus, they have not been particularly attentive to their MOU responsibilities" (Narrative Report, 2001).

The Structural Pest Control Commission (the State Lead Agency) folks were pretty unhappy when this observation went to the USEPA. The fact is, these good ol' boys did not want to do the work or upset the exterminators whom they were supposed to regulate. However, they couldn't have it both ways — protect their exterminators and take credit for implementing real IPM. They refused to attend any training sessions. It was pretty obvious they were trying to talk the walk rather than walk the walk, and my team was pretty damn' offended by their free rider attitude. Fortunately, the folks up in USEPA Region 9 also were fed up with their behavior and this incident resulted in a this-is-how-the-cow-ate-the-cabbage talk. Soon after, Carl Martin assumed more control of this program from the Commission and became one of our major champions for school IPM. In all fairness to the Commission's administration, this program was something new and different. It was perceived as a political risk and a possibly time-consuming unfunded mandate. I understood this but admittedly was not too sympathetic — been there, done that. I can happily report that in the years since the pilot program, most of these people seem more comfortable with and supportive of IPM.

The school administration and Extension specialists were providing leadership beyond our expectations. The school business manager was aggressively pursuing statewide implementation by developing a School IPM Symposium for the state's association of school business managers, and an aggressive PR program. Dawn was successful in obtaining state funding for an IPM training program from the State Lead Agency. Mike Lindsey developed and utilized considerable expertise in implementing IPM in the pilot schools and was the key component in our training program, especially regarding the educational component for the staff and teachers

Please let me caution you. Progress did not happen overnight. It took months of handholding by our team to assure school administrators and especially staff that they could implement IPM within the confines of their current job responsibilities and budgets. Change is tough. Influencing attitudes and changing behavior requires a lot of well-thought-out communication. Fact sheets and websites alone will not suffice in this situation. They help reinforce the message, but it is in this implementation stage that change agents must get their hands dirty.

Mike was always getting dirty, just as one would expect from an old-fashioned, cotton IPM man. The very pleasant surprise was the extent to which the University of Arizona urban entomologists became involved. Dawn developed newsletters and fact sheets, but also made sure she was involved with the hands-on training that was so critical. She even came up with the idea of having the Arizona Department of Game and Fish release owls for rodent control. Dawn patiently instructed custodians on how to identify conducive conditions for indoor and outdoor pests. The timing was right. These Extension entomologists got involved with something meaningful and interesting before their careers sank into mundane functions of providing for "traditional" Extension customers.

John Carter and Stan Peterson were able to conduct an excellent analysis of the true cost of pest management for the district. Like the vast majority of districts in the country, Kyrene did not delineate pest management as a line item in the overall operations budget. Thus, in the initial analysis it was apparent that the district ascribed a nominal budget for the contractual cost of pest management in 25 schools. Upon further analysis, it was determined that the actual annual cost of pest management (contract + extra pesticide applications + administrative hours) was approximately three times the original contractor estimate. This finding illustrates what our team has found in all program areas. Traditional pest management is no more cost effective than a quality IPM program, is less efficient at addressing short- and long-term pest problems/complaints and unnecessarily exposes children and adult inhabitants of the school to pesticides. The model was working!

Reinforcing the message that "you can do this and it is the right thing" with pest monitoring and economic data really did the trick. Stan and his staff were beginning to believe. Our next step was to get Stan and his bosses to decide that they wanted to continue and expand the program. Below were my recommendations to the USEPA and implementation team for this next step:

1) Begin administrative transition to district-wide implementation. Several options are available to the administration:
   a. internalize the IPM program via training and designate an IPM Coordinator (it is particularly important that this individual obtain training far beyond current state certification, have an administratively approved job

      description and receive performance reviews that evaluate success operating a COMPLETE IPM program);

    b. develop a partnership with a competent pest management professional for purposes of facility assessment and pest problem resolution, to work with the designated district administrative staff; and

    c. contract with a pest management professional to provide a full-service program. This option will be successful only under rigorous contract specifications AND an MOU outlining the district's responsibilities for communication and structural/sanitary remediation.

2) It is strongly recommended that a more structured communication plan be prepared by the state program partners for program status and coordination.

3) Develop and send out a press release regarding the success and expansion of this program.

4) The state partners and the PESP team should develop a plan for statewide implementation. Currently, it appears that the most daunting problem facing the implementation of IPM in schools statewide is the LACK of identified, competent and willing pest management professionals to address the technical aspects of this type of program. It is strongly recommended that program partners meet and address this issue BEFORE proceeding.

5) It is strongly recommended that the USEPA develop a team approach (Regional Manager, Pest Management Professional, Independent Coordinator and School Administrator Peers) to accelerate the adoption of IPM in schools nationally. Further, USEPA should use existing or earmarked funds to appoint and support a national school IPM coordinator to coordinate the leadership of transferable models, and expand those models to other states. (Lame, 2001)

LESSON 1: It takes a team and teamwork.

We needed to develop a team approach (a program coordinator, someone from the feds to help with agency barriers, a Pest Management Professional, an on-site coordinator and a "peer" school administrator) to accelerate the adoption of IPM in schools nationally. It makes no sense to re-invent the team in every state. This is not a one-man show. There are too many aspects to manage — technical, economical, logistical, political and public relations. It requires know-how and support. We all were hanging our reputations out there and were not sure the outcome would be pleasant. The traditional opposition to IPM was sharpening its knives, and we all had day jobs. Finally, funding from Cooperative Extension was non-existent for school IPM and damn' little was available from USEPA. We needed to get the most bang for our bucks.

Results

Six months into our test program the Kyrene School District indicated it intended to expand the pilot program to ALL schools in the district. This decision was based on the enthusiasm of the pilot school staff and district administrators' realization that they had experienced a decrease in pesticide use of more than 90% and a reduction of pest complaints by more than 85%. As decisionmakers, they had been able to incorporate IPM into their existing management without increasing their workload, while significantly decreasing pesticide use.

My final report to the USEPA about our change agents in Arizona:

"The University of Arizona Department of Entomology (Drs. Baker and Gouge) and Cooperative Extension Administration (Dr. Jim Christensen) have proven to be incredible resources for this type of program. The remarkable success of the current program is in large part due to their dedicated personnel and community-based philosophy. The model used and improved by this team has extreme potential to increase the spread of IPM in schools throughout the southwestern United States. It is strongly recommended that the State and the USEPA recognize these entities and individuals for their efforts to implement IPM in schools and to reduce the risk of unnecessary exposure to pesticides by children. Further, that the state partners and the PESP team develop a plan for statewide implementation" (Lame, 2001).

For Mike Lindsey (our on-site coordinator), who was required to:
- Conduct bi-weekly inspections (with documentation) of each pilot school for the duration of the program.
- Attend all training sessions.
- Attend all school technical inspections conducted by the PESP Partner
- Educate the school personnel with regard to pests, pest prevention and program status during each scheduled visit.
- Maintain on-call availability for pest complaints or emergencies.

- Demonstrate a willingness to coordinate activities with other states (MOU, Appendix D).

> [I said] "Mike Lindsey has developed and utilized considerable expertise implementing IPM in the pilot schools and has been the key component in our training program — especially regarding the educational component for the staff and teachers. In particular, Mr. Lindsey has organized a successful scorpion IPM program in heretofore chronically infested areas. Further, he has conducted numerous presentations to the teachers and students regarding the benefits of arthropod pests –"not all bugs are bad". Not enough can be said about Mr. Lindsey's incredible communication and teaching techniques. A real pro."

Like any good scorpion-loving entomologist, Mike keeps the Giant Hairy Desert scorpion as a pet (yes, he is still married). So, he got excited about finding a large population of scorpions at our problem school and wanted to "fix 'em good". Based on his nighttime monitoring for scorpions (that is when they hunt for prey), Mike discovered they had made the cinder block wall at one edge of the school property their home. Each hollow block was a "scorpion condo". Stan had the wall stuccoed, thereby eliminating habitat. This simple and fairly inexpensive mechanical control reduced the scorpion problem by 90%, and Mike's "scorpion wall" became a much-talked-about example of how mechanical control works in southwestern schools.

Mike inspires people. A teacher who worked with him at the middle school developed a math curriculum based on insect monitoring. Science teachers and their students followed Stan around the school just to see what pests his monitoring traps had snared. He inspired Dawn to experiment with the use of soil amendments, which increased the permeability of the playground soils. Why? Because these soils are flood-irrigated and the standing water breeds mosquitoes. Even before the West Nile Virus scare of 2002 Dawn (quite keen on medical entomology) was concerned about standing water and artificial lakes in the Phoenix area. This little experiment to help water soak into the ground worked! Not only was mosquito habitat reduced, but so were fire ants in the grassy areas. It was cultural control at its best.

After the initial three-school pilot program in 2000, Kyrene School District expanded its integrated pest management program to all 26 district schools. This reduced the exposure of more than 20,000 districts students, faculty and staff to possibly dangerous pesticides and pests. Stan chose a combination of options A and B, utilizing his grounds supervisor as an IPM coordinator and contracting with an independent Pest Management Professional to conduct school assessments and give advice. And we developed a national team of implementers that included the folks from the University of Arizona, Structural Pest Control Board, Monroe County Community School Corporation, Kyrene, Bobby Corrigan and USEPA Regions 5 and 9.

LESSON 2: Help your state implementation team expand its political base.

I have preached for years that if Cooperative Extension would concentrate more on schools it could expand its political base way beyond agribusiness or the pest control industry. The same goes for State Lead Agencies and even school administrators. Instead of limiting yourself to what was, look at what is. And "what is" are parents. Getting good press and awards for school boards (elected by parents, not just farmers and pesticide folks) and university departments whose budgets are allocated by legislators (elected by parents, not just farmers and pesticide folks) expands the political base for our team members and gives them some protection (that years before, I had lacked) to "do the right thing".

Epilogue

USEPA subsequently recognized the school district and the University of Arizona, Department of Entomology for their IPM efforts. In the fall of 2002, and after continued successful implementation, Kyrene School District, the state and the university were honored by the National Foundation for IPM Education with a plaque during a press conference. This program was to become a model to other schools in the Southwest, including those on the Navajo Indian Reservation.

Chapter Eight - Expanding the Model in Alabama

I attended graduate school in Auburn, Alabama, and absolutely loved it. Three years out of college I applied to university graduate programs in entomology at the University of Arizona and Auburn University. I figured I couldn't get into Auburn because it was a Southern Ivy League school, but believed I could probably afford to go to Arizona because I was a resident of the state. I was working on a temporary appointment with the USDA Animal, Plant Health Inspection Service (APHIS) pink bollworm and rangeland caterpillar management programs during the day and as a doorman at a large bar in Tempe at night. I knew if I didn't attend graduate school I'd be a field grunt for the rest of my career.

The University of Arizona turned me down, so I went to talk to George Ware (Entomology Department Head at the University of Arizona) to ask why. George asked me what I was doing at the time and I told him. He was pretty interested in my job as a bouncer and not too impressed with my achievement test scores. He told me if I worked hard enough I could become the best bouncer in Arizona. That was the end of the interview. In later years, I found that George was a real character and that his response to my future plans was "just George". The funny thing is that when I finished my degree at Auburn, George hired me to become an IPM coordinator with his department. I guess that was because Auburn was one of the best applied entomology departments in the country. George didn't even recall who I was... just that I had "trained" at Auburn.

The department at Auburn was small, but very interactive and friendly. Southern hospitality is real, and as a student of the department, I found a wonderful place to live and learn for the next three years. Dr. Max Bass convinced American Cyanamid chemical company to support my research on the Red Imported Fire Ant. I did some of the product formulation work on a product still used today called Amdro®. My professors were great teachers and mentors. One of them was Dr. Mike Williams who taught me how to collect and identify hundreds of families of insects — a critical skill for a field entomologist. In 1999, I called Mike and asked him if he would be interested in working with me to expand IPM in schools with our model. He invited me down to talk about it.

The Players

Change Agents

According to the grant that John Carter and I proposed, we would extend the IPM model to Arizona and Alabama at the same time. Our implementation plan and materials were virtually identical — the same MOU, training, assessment and evaluation procedures and tools. Soon after my initial visit to Tempe I met with Mike's proposed team in Auburn: Fudd Graham, at the time a doctoral student (yes, he did graduate, and we call him Dr. Fudd), a research associate in charge of the state's fire ant program, and the Extension IPM Coordinator, Mark Rumph. They would be our entomology department leads.

Fudd had been a licensed Pest Control Operator so he had down-and-dirty experience with most of the pests we would be dealing with. He was just about as good as you can get when it comes to managing the Red Imported Fire Ant. He eventually became part of our national team and has been instrumental in moving the implementation of real school IPM in the South. Mark was a real politician, and with a growing family and little training in entomology would leave our program shortly before it concluded. He grew up in Auburn and had contacts with Auburn City Schools.

Our Indiana team, Bobby Corrigan, John Carter, Jerry Jochim and I, drove down in the spring to conduct initial training and assess the economics, policies and technical situation (pests, pesticides and conducive conditions). If I remember correctly, Bobby said it was one of his career highpoints to spend nine hours in the car listening to me opine on various world problems....or maybe the longest night of his life – I forget.

The School District

Unlike Kyrene, where I made initial contact with the school district, Mark lined up all the folks in the Auburn system. As with Kyrene, the administration was willing to work with us as long as it didn't cost anything. As with Monroe County schools and the "university town" relationship, they were fairly trusting of Mark and Fudd. When I first met with them they seemed to like the idea that I had lived in Auburn for a while. We would be working with Jim Divinney, the Assistant Superintendent, and his custodial and kitchen supervisors. They agreed to work within perimeters of the MOU I required, and we were set to start in the late spring.

The district was about a third the size of Monroe County or Kyrene, and represented what one might find in a small city. Auburn had seven schools with about 4,500 students. One or two of the schools were pretty old, but most were built in the '70s and '80s. They were in reasonable repair. Other than size, Auburn also had a different management culture than Kyrene or Monroe County. It seemed to be more formal on the administrative side, and maybe because it was smaller, the school principals carried a lot of weight. Further, many of the teachers in the pilot schools, kept Raid® in their classrooms, felt pesticide use was a good thing and at first were not happy about alternatives. Our pilot schools were pretty typical. We usually like to have one high school, a middle school and an elementary school. At Auburn we had the high school and two elementary schools.

The Pest Control Operators

This was the first district where we were able to actually work with the outside contractor (I have already mentioned Richard Lumpkin). At that time, Richard worked for a long- established local pest control firm. To his credit the owner (who was already giving the schools a discounted price because he was part of the community) told Richard to work with us. Initially, Richard was very cooperative, but not too happy. He viewed our program as a threat and as extra work. We found out he had to work with us all day on our training and assessments and then go service his accounts. Richard is a no-nonsense kind of guy. He did not feel our program was necessary but he was very candid about his feelings. When asked what he did for pest control, he said he applied pesticides to the outside perimeter of the school buildings to prevent pests. He really did not have much knowledge about which chemicals or the history. However, he later would spend hours of his personal time recovering historical information about pesticide use for us. Prior to our program he was told to spray and he did — a lot.

Richard followed us around on our technical assessments. At first, he lingered at the back of our entourage and didn't pay much attention. However, when we started turning up German cockroaches in places he hadn't considered (like the fish tank lamps in the biology classroom

– warm, wet and containing bits of food that never made it to the water – roach paradise), he started listening a bit. We always make it a point to talk about what can be done to manage pests better, rather than whose fault it is. While I do fault some people in this book, I do not feel it appropriate or fair to fault the people on the "front lines" for something they were required to do or were never informed about a better way. Richard is smart. He knew what he had been doing to control pests, and now he was learning what made sense. We showed him pest-conducive conditions and how to use monitoring traps and pesticide baits. We were able to prove that pesticides do not prevent structural pests. Most of all, we empowered him with sufficient knowledge, ability and authority to become a valued partner with the school district in managing its pests. Fudd recently told me he heard Richard, when told by a teacher to spray his classroom, tell that customer if he wanted someone to spray, they should get someone else. This is the difference between a pest management professional and an exterminator. This is power that a dearly few pest management professionals are accorded by school administrators.

Pests and Conducive Conditions

One of the reasons I loved going to school in the South was the region has great bugs — warm and wet. All you have to do is add food and poof! – bugs. Alabama has a scorpion that is smaller and less poisonous than those in Arizona. There also are Brown Recluse spiders and snakes. All of these could be found in and around the Auburn schools. Internally, we encountered pretty much the same pest complex as we had in Indiana and Arizona — mice, cockroaches, houseflies, filth flies, stinging wasps, ants and spiders. However, Auburn did have one different kind of roach. The Smokeybrown looks very similar to the American cockroach but has slightly different coloring and behavior, which makes it more prone to infesting buildings. The South also has the Red Imported Fire Ant. This pest has displaced many of the ant species one normally would find around schools, it has huge colonies, and of course they sting more readily and purposefully than other ants. I cannot tell you how many times I have been stung by fire ants. In the South if you spend lot of time outdoors you get stung by fire ants, and if you research them you get stung a lot more. I personally find their sting to be painful, but much less so than that of a bee, wasp or even the Harvester Ants in the West (which almost never sting, but have some nasty toxin). They are definitely a nuisance to homeowners and school children, and their mounds can be damaging to machinery, but they're dangerous only to those allergic or too infirm to move away.

115

The most severe pest in our Auburn pilot schools was the German cockroach (known as water bugs in Alabama). All the schools had some level of German cockroach infestation. Fortunately, this species is easily eliminated with IPM, but not very well controlled with sprays or aerosol application of pesticides. We found them everywhere — in classrooms, pantries, kitchens, locker rooms, gymnasium, custodial closets, and as usual, the teachers' lounge. They particularly liked the area surrounding the deep fryer in the high school kitchen, and as mentioned, the biology classrooms. The Smokeybrowns were less common but more persistent. All the schools had fire ants on their playgrounds and some problems with them entering food serving areas (these ants love grease). We found lots of fruit flies and wasps. One school reported that the mice were so bad they were dropping out of the ceilings onto desks and people. So much for prevention through the application of pesticides.

In general, the primary reason these schools had so many pests stemmed from the degree of sanitation. We found it to be below that of Monroe County and Kyrene. The school with the best sanitation, Dean Road Elementary, had the fewest pest problems. Not coincidentally, this school's principal was a real communicator, and the head custodian really took ownership of the entire facility. Throughout the district, trash management (particularly the dumpsters) was sloppy, and the kitchens were cleaned only superficially.

One example of the poor communication and sanitation levels occurred at the high school. In the kitchen an "overlooked" box of potatoes was rotting under the sink and serving as a breeding substrate for thousands of fruit flies. As we find in most other districts, the kitchen staff relied on custodial staff to clean up after them. While this is okay, better communication was needed between these staff members. With the rotting potatoes, I suspect the custodial staff did not want to discard the box because they knew it "belonged" to the kitchen staff, so neither discussed the problem. Another example typical of many schools is that coaches or band directors have custodians or maintenance staff apply fairly toxic materials to the playing fields whenever they think it appropriate — independent of any pest management consultation or education. Coaches rule. Ask any facilities manager. At Auburn, diazinon was commonly applied to playing fields for fire ant control, and the 20-pound pesticide bag was kept in the music department.

How the Program Progressed

As usual, it took a while for things to get off the ground. Our most significant problems seemed related to communication. Auburn was very hierarchical when it came to changing procedures. The custodial and kitchen supervisors wouldn't make any changes unless they were approved by the supervisor's office. Whereas this centralized management situation works IF a decisionmaker in the supervisor's office is informed and willing to take action, make changes such as recommendations to remediate pest-conducive conditions or cessation of chemical pesticide use without approval - otherwise the program will grind to a halt.

LESSON 3: Develop a direct line of communication with the decision maker.

Because I had agreed to work through the Extension IPM Coordinator, communication was at times not very efficient. The middle man approach to communication works only if a rigid schedule is in place to assure the transfer of information. Further, at Auburn there was a bit of a turf problem between the Extension Coordinator and the on-site coordinator. Thus, I believe that one must always formally designate a line of authority for coordinating a multi-jurisdictional program — or walk away from it. Fortunately, in this case, Mike Williams came to the rescue and we got back on track. Mark concentrated on getting information to and from kitchen and custodial staff. Fudd worked extensively with Richard, training him to recognize conducive conditions and use bait for roaches and fire ants instead of more toxic materials. Over time, Mark and Fudd began to coordinate efforts. In fact, one of the improvements we made with the Auburn program was to invite the Alabama team to Arizona for mid-term evaluations. This not only allowed more training for the change agents, but also increased the esprit de corps of our national implementation team.

In general, the program went much the same as at Kyrene. We conducted two training programs for staff and distributed several newsletters. Richard proved to be an enthusiastic convert and donated significant time and materials (monitors and cockroach bait). Bobby and I conducted the initial and midterm pest management evaluations. Though he had other fire ant responsibilities, Fudd (our on-site IPM coordinator) really got into the program. As a true convert he wrote, "I vaguely remember someone mentioning that they might be able to get me a copy of the URBAN IPM BIBLE written in a New York accent by Bobby Corrigan. I have been contacted to teach the group of Pest Management Professionals. A little reference material would be greatly appreciated, if you can round me up one" (Graham, 2001). It makes an evangelical IPM guy feel pretty good when folks start asking for reading material. Fudd conducted and submitted inspection/treatment reports each month. These evaluations demonstrated that the school system complied with recommendations to improve sanitation and exclusion practices which were also integrated with chemical bait for cockroaches. The evaluations Fudd gave us showed a radical decline in pest populations.

Not surprisingly, the State Lead Agency did not become very involved with the program and did not attend any of the training sessions. I suspect there were some of the same problems that we saw with Arizona — the fear of change, unfunded extra work and of angering the industry. However, I also must admit it was more difficult for the State Lead Agency folks to travel to Auburn from Montgomery. The guys I worked with seemed very supportive, but just didn't know how much they could risk on this program. This, too, has changed over the years.

The Results

The results of pest management in our pilot schools were almost identical to those in the Kyrene program. The schools experienced a 90% reduction in pesticide application and an 85% reduction in pest complaints. In the fall of 2001, six months into the program, the Auburn City Schools decided to expand the pilot program to all city schools, including their preschool program. This decision was based on the enthusiasm of pilot school principals and district administrators. As with the Kyrene program, once the decisionmakers realized they could incorporate IPM into their existing management without increasing their costs, significantly decrease pesticide use and take back the schools from the water bugs, they were convinced to adopt IPM. Most importantly, said one of the school principals, "We are doing this because it is the right thing for the children."

LESSON 4: Play nice with the principal.

This principal was Dr. Nancy Golson. Surprisingly, she turned out to be the activist in the school system. Site-based management is a term used by school officials. It means that the principal is the boss of the school site. While custodial supervisors (who work for the facilities manager, who works for the superintendent) get to hire fire and determine policies and procedures for cleaning, cooking and fixing, the principal has the last say on what gets done and whether or not it is satisfactory to the boss.

We usually find that school principals we work with (we try to talk to all of them) just don't take the time to talk to us. I don't know if they are too busy, don't care or view us as lowly exterminators. I admit I still have a problem with principals stemming from several painful experiences I had as a student. To this day I still get nervous sitting on that bench in front of the principal's office. Fortunately, in every program we have conducted, one principal has been able to see the value — or maybe is just plain interested in bugs (who could blame them?). Nancy was interested from the start. Maybe it was the high level of professional courtesy that one finds in the South, but she met with us and promised cooperation. Indeed, she was the principal, who along with her head custodian, Mr. Penny, implemented our program so effectively that other principals in the district were convinced to adopt IPM. I understand that she touted our program at a principals' meeting. This is gold! If the principals want it and it doesn't cost the district anything, it will happen. Ironically, as can happen, the district did adopt IPM, but within a year decided to contract with a low-bid pesticides contractor. Richard was out and someone who said he could do IPM was in. I hear that when Nancy found this out there was a "school yard" discussion with district decisionmakers. Evidently, Nancy quickly educated her partners at the district and real IPM prevailed. Nancy has become one of our national advisors and still educates me once in a while.

Auburn City Schools and Auburn University have since been recognized by the USEPA and the National Foundation for IPM Education for their contributions toward protecting the environmental health of the children of Alabama. I believe Mike Williams put it correctly when he described his school community as one that "thinks with their heads and commits with their hearts". Thanks to Fudd, the State Lead Agency (Alabama Department of Agriculture and Industry) in Montgomery seems interested enough to participate in and support more IPM models in Alabama. The remarkable success of the Auburn program is in large part due to its dedicated personnel and community-based philosophy of Auburn University. The model used and improved by this team has great potential to increase the spread of IPM in schools throughout the southern United States. Florida is our current project and it's working beyond expectations. Unfortunately, after the glow of success in Alabama, we lost the next gamble in Las Vegas.

Chapter Nine - Gambling in Las Vegas

In the fall of 2000, Charles Moses with the Nevada Department of Agriculture approached the Clark County School District in Las Vegas, seeking to have the district pilot our Monroe IPM Model. Chuck's department is the State Lead Agency authorized by the USEPA to implement the Federal Insecticide, Fungicide, Rodenticide Act – FIFRA. Chuck believed a mandate for school IPM was inevitable and was busting his butt to be out front on this issue — both for the schools and his own department's sake. We viewed Clark County as particularly important and challenging, as it is one of the largest and fastest growing school districts in the country. It includes the majority of schools in the state of Nevada. Demonstrating IPM in this type of school environment would create a model for large school districts throughout the U.S. and make Clark County a national peer leader for national implementation of IPM in schools. Clark County was receptive, but as you will see, not really prepared to commit to even a pilot program. This project went screwy from the beginning and I have since kicked myself repeatedly for wasting precious time and money available for implementing IPM in schools. However, my Monroe IPM Model partners have reminded me many times that we learned more with this program than in all of our others combined. In this chapter I will attempt to build a detailed case for how one might avoid costly mistakes.

CONTACT

Our initial meeting to convince Clark County School District took place in October, 2000. This was a fairly large meeting of district

120

officials, pest control operators, the State Lead Agency rep, a Cooperative Agent, Bobby Corrigan and me. The district officials were receptive, but indecisive. Keep in mind that this is the sixth largest school system in the nation and is the fastest growing district in the country — approximately 280 schools. As usual, pest management is a back burner issue. As far as pest management was concerned, the district really didn't know what it was doing, how much it was spending or why it should change.

A nationally recognized pest control company's commercial division (which from now on I will now call "the firm") handled pest management for all the school kitchens. Their manager professed to be fully into IPM for the school pest management program. "The firm" evinced a willingness to work with us, but when asked not to pre-bait, it launched the standard arguments. I was very clear that our program does not use preventative treatments. They were not happy and went into the Health Department inspection scare tactic — "a single pest will cause a violation..." Be advised, I was uncharacteristically nice and inclusive with these folks. However, I will not go along with any preventive treatments for pilot programs. We advised the district administrators that the no-treatment-without-consultation/permission clause would be in effect with our MOU. I requested that all pre-baiting in the pilot schools (scheduled for the end of summer) be suspended, as well as any treatment for termites.

For the most part, it was an informative meeting. After Bobby and I presented the logic for implementing IPM and what our program consisted of, everyone seemed pretty comfortable with trying a pilot program. In fact, we actually sent Stan Peterson up from Kyrene to talk to the Clark County School District folks about his experience with our model and any concerns they might have. I found it interesting that at this initial meeting the Cooperative Extension Agent from Clark County was late, didn't say a word and never showed his face again. Obviously, the university would not be participating as a change agent in Nevada.

I should have known there were problems when it took another eight months to move to the next step, but Chuck convinced a local reporter to do a story on the impending program and forced Clark County School District to get off the stick. The next summer John Carter, Jerry Jochim and I met with Chuck and the administrators at Clark County School District to finalize the Memorandum of Understanding, develop the pilot schools plan and conduct a preliminary assessment of each pilot school. This meeting got off to a rocky start. The district officials seemed to want the project, but were obviously in no hurry to kick it off. They were restructuring, and not in the mood for any more changes. Their huge administration had the same problem our other districts had: facilities staff controlled facilities and academic staff controlled academics (teachers, students, etc.). While the facilities (operations) folks were getting their heads around this, no one brought in the principals, assistant principals, etc. to partner up. It was a warning sign and a lesson we were still learning. I definitely got the feeling that the administrators I was dealing with wanted a free, warm and fuzzy program they could toss the parents, but were unwilling to really work at it. In fact, on the way to our meeting, Chuck informed me that he was unaware of any choice of pilot schools or that anyone had talked to any principal. In the first five minutes of the meeting we found that the assistant superintendent was not coming, and that the same district administrators from our initial meeting were at the table. I expected a "sorry, not interested" response, or at least waffling to occur, and was ready to walk. Our strategy was to let them know we assumed all was ready to go. My words were: "I am ready to get dirty looking for your bugs today." At that point I perceived a major lack of eye contact with those I hoped were my partners-to-be.

Just when I figured it was not going to happen and Chuck was beginning to blow, the administrator of operations smiled and said, "Oh, we have the pilot schools picked out!" At that point her minions began bobbing their heads and asking if we were ready to visit the pilot schools (which we believe were picked about 10 minutes before the meeting began). Sighs of relief! Chuck mumbled (he was just building up a good head of steam). Of course, I said, we were good to go, and I proudly produced my new bug inspecting equipment belt with multiple flashlights.

I always ask the decisionmaker from the school district we are trying to work with, "Give us your schools with the worst bug problems". In this case, I really don't know how the pilot schools were chosen, but they definitely had pest problems. We were taken to Rancho High School, vintage circa 1930; PA Diskin Elementary, circa 1980; and Ed Von Tobel Middle School; circa 1964. Another school, Crestwood Elementary, originally had been picked, but was nixed because it was set to be taken over by a private firm and would not be workable. (Hence our suspicion about the hasty pilot schools designation that morning.) An interesting if not ironic footnote is that the Edison folks who were to become the private trustees of these public schools had run into severe financial problems. Clark County School District had more and bigger problems than roaches in its kitchens.

We further developed our implementation team at this point. John Carter immediately went to work obtaining stats regarding size, population, custodial load, etc. and would be consulting with Stan at Kyrene. Jerry assisted Bobby and me with our technical assessments. One of our big problems was that we had no on-site coordinators. We brought in Lyn Hawkins from California to handle this role. Lyn's work on IPM goes back to before it was called IPM. He had recently retired from the Cal EPA where he worked with the implementation of IPM in schools and agriculture. Lyn is a great educator. Of course Chuck Moses was on board from the state, and he was already working with Mary Grisier from USEPA Region 9. Mike Wallace from the National Foundation for IPM Education joined us as an advisor and facilitator for developing plans we hoped would become the national model for implementing IPM in schools.

LESSON 5: Make sure your On-Site IPM Coordinator is on-site.

Lyn did a great job as our on-site coordinator. He visited the schools at least monthly, communicated often and presented educational material at staff training sessions. However, I believe you need to have in this position someone who is part of the community — if not local, at least state community. This allows for better understanding of the technical and political situations. Also, it allows for a more on-call availability that provides both real and perceived comfort to the school pest managers.

What we were walking into.

Pest management in Clark County School District falls under three administrations: two (Grounds and Facilities) in Operations, and one in Food Services:

Grounds (landscape, playgrounds and playing fields) was under the direction of a well-trained professional. He had been switching landscaping to indigenous varieties of plants, with the exception of playing fields, for most of the newer schools. However, the older schools' landscapes were grass and trees (probably from Hoboken, NJ) that required a lot of water. Fortunately, flood-type irrigation had been eliminated district-wide. *Unfortunately*, drought-stressed landscape is prone to pest infestation. Major pesticide use revolved around using Roundup® on weeds. In our initial meeting I explained to the groundskeepers that Lyn Hawkins had a lot of experience with the California weeds situation and could work with them. I also explained that Grounds would be addressed later in the pilot program rather than sooner. Africanized Bees were a serious (though not major) problem in this district. Clark County School District contracted with "bee master" Rodney Mehring, Jr., to handle this problem. Rodney was present at our initial meeting and very cooperative. He is very active in the National Pest Management Association and was interested in our descriptions of what professional pest managers should look like, and when and how to use them (from my fact sheet "What is and What is not IPM in schools", Appendix A).

School facilities (classrooms, auditoriums, concession stands, school offices, etc.) were under the direction of the custodial supervisor and the maintenance/planning supervisor. The custodial supervisor was pretty squared away with the bureaucracy and seemed supportive. Pest problems were referred by work order from a school employee (teacher, coach, secretary, etc.) to Operations, then back to principals for approval and NOTIFICATION, then finally to the licensed Pest Control Operator. They actually used the word "spraying" in their outdated notification form.

The district had one licensed Pest Control Operator. He was poorly trained, but enthusiastic. He worked at night and had virtually no contact with the referring entities. He applied pesticides when told to by custodians, principals, or teachers. He did communicate with school principals when he found generally pest-conducive conditions. However, he had no authority, was at the bottom of the totem pole and didn't have much training to communicate with his clients, anyway.

In the months preceding our program, this "in-house exterminator" substituted indoor spraying for what he called baits. Near as I could figure from our conversations, he was using Max Force® granules indoors upon request and chlorpyriphos granules on the perimeter (outside walls and doorways) throughout "problem schools" periodically. He didn't utilize monitoring stations. Treatments were broadcast (versus crack and crevasse). Unbelievably, chlorpyriphos granules were found three feet from the external walls, and at times covered, lost or forgotten lunch boxes and reusable water bottles that students left behind. Many dead sewer roaches (American cockroaches) lay in un-swept internal areas.

On the good side, the school system was very serious about implementing a new energy management program (due to California "brown-out" fears) and told me most of my suggested structural modifications were what they needed to undertake, anyway. The trash bags had good mil specs, which meant they were less likely to break open and attract pests when thrown into the dumpster. In some ways it looked as though some of the major components for mechanical control and monitoring were in place.

Major internal pests included sewer roaches, mice, spiders (mostly Black Widows), ants, silverfish and some flies. I did find evidence of a German Cockroach infestation in the middle school. Interestingly, the same school presented a "no-see-um" (biting gnat) problem in one classroom. These probably bred after recent rains, in mud adjacent neighborhood construction. No pest logs were in use.

It was obvious there was no conscious effort by the administration responsible for pest management to implement IPM at the schools we visited. Their in-house guy was a bait jockey at best (he since has moved on to working as your friendly home exterminator), but he seemed to be motivated. Our challenge was to convert him, with the blessing of his bosses, to a pest manager through training, authorization and scheduling (his visitation schedule made him invisible). This training is all about the conversion from scheduled killer to educator/diagnostician. As we had experienced with all of the school districts with which we have worked, he had problems with teachers owning and using Raid® to combat real and perceived bug problems. Did I mention they still fogged for lice in some of these schools? It's a totally worthless and possibly dangerous practice, as lice don't live overnight away from their human food sources.

Kitchens used for food preparation or service were under the direction of the Food Service Director. Food was prepared and sent to the elementary schools. As I mentioned, a nationally recognized pest control company's commercial division handled pest management for all kitchens. They serviced the high schools and middle schools once per month and the elementary schools twice a year. Their manager attended our initial meeting and professed to be fully into IPM for the school program. Their existing program consisted of pre-baiting all kitchens two times per year for roaches, ants and crickets and using residual chemical insecticide applications on the exterior entries of the kitchens. They used monitors and containerized mechanical trap or bait stations for mice.

As you will come to see, pest conditions in the kitchens were fair to poor. No way was this firm implementing a full-scale IPM program in these kitchens. First, how can one begin to address a monitoring situation in a pest-vulnerable area by monitoring only twice per year? I suppose this was the reason for pre-baiting all kitchens. Second, preventive treatments (particularly exterior) are not part of an IPM program. Third, inspections indicated little or no communication (either the fault of the school or the technician) regarding conducive conditions for pests or pest-related health violations.

Examples of poor pest management in the kitchen areas were old bait stations improperly placed (vertical substrates – walls), undated monitors, dead mice (mummified) in mechanical traps, leaky commercial rodent-bait stations, rat poison purchased at retail outlets with translocatable pellets (pretty, bright green pellets that could look like candy to children), unsanitary conditions and structural decomposition. Some of the pest problems were related to the abundance of insect carcasses accessible for periods of time — again, not necessarily the responsibility of the technician, but a direct result of baiting without communicating the proper cause-and-effect relationship of sanitation and pests to the custodial and kitchen staff.

I sure wish that just once we could walk into a program where the contractor who swears he utilizes IPM is really performing even close to our standards. I don't object to these guys saying they are progressive pest managers or even exterminators (because that might be all they are being asked or paid to do by the district), but that is a far cry from real IPM. I strongly recommended that the technicians from "the firm" who were handling the pilots attend both the training program and walk-through training that Bobby and I conducted. I was looking forward to "the firm" attempting to work on the same page as us on this program — hope springs eternal.

Rancho High School was definitely the worst of the pilot schools we worked with. It's old, neglected, used as a training ground for new administrators and as a last duty post for those near retirement. It is an inner-city school, smaller than Bloomington High School, but with twice the number of students, and fewer custodial staff. It kinda reminded me of Auburn High School. It had a lot of vending machines (a.k.a., "bug supermarkets"), holes in walls, old concession stands, a new gym and an old gym (scary place — Bobby had to hold Lyn's hand just to get him in the door).

The custodial staff actually liked the feral cats because they killed mice. Nearly everyone hated pigeons, but they weren't numerous. The school had discontinued use of all bottom lockers because it could not keep the Black Widows from nesting in them. Major pests included mice, American Cockroaches, the aforementioned Black Widow spiders, and ants (Harvester ants, Southern fire ants and Argentine ants). Underground conduits ran throughout the school. We opened one and found adult and immature American Roaches and Indian House Crickets in abundance. We knew that a chemical pesticide component would be needed and that the in-house licensed Pest Control Operator would have to learn to use a bait gun. Bait guns (look like a miniature caulking gun) are a much more effective way to apply a relatively safe chemical option, as opposed to the types of baits and application the operator was then using.

The staff lounge in the cafeteria appeared reasonably clean, and vending machines were okay, but the cove base and serving station were poorly sealed, garbage cans were full and mouse droppings were obvious in front of the microwave oven. The cafeteria itself had 18 vending machines and inadequate door sweeps, and the storage/utility room in the cafeteria had popcorn and fixings on the floor with lots of mouse poop and poor mop storage. We found a dying American Cockroach on the floor being eaten by a horde of ants. I bring this up because I noticed the dead roaches throughout the school seemed to act as a food source/attractant to ants.

The kitchen was old, trashed, peeling paint and had greasy floors. Dead roaches or roach parts were the least of the health violations in this facility. "The firm's" sticky trap monitors were scattered throughout — trashed, undated and misplaced. "The firm's" mouse trap was last monitored three months prior to our inspection. Some 30-40 dead American Roaches littered the floor, nymphs of the same were present (indicating an infestation), a roach bait station was located on the wall (improper vertical placement), and a 2-inch "mouse run" extended behind all ground level cupboards. The pantry area had decent shelving, but also had a hole chewed in the wall at ground level, with lots of mouse poop. "The firm's" mechanical mousetrap contained a mummified mouse. Their mouse bait station had a disintegrating bait tab leaking from it. At least two retail bait stations were evident in this room, and they contained those pretty, green pellets — rat poison. Professional pest managers didn't use these stations, which indicated two big problems: Kitchen personnel were using a registered poison inconsistent with the label instructions (pretty green poison pellets near food being served to children); and they were not removed or reported by "the firm". I consider this lack of action highly unprofessional. Supposedly "the firm" knew what connotes good and safe pest management. Finally, there was evidence of a current mouse infestation. The baits weren't cutting it because so much other food was around for the mice to dine on.

The kitchen loading dock had a dirty grease bin close to the door and a filthy area with milk carton containers stacked against the wall. Doors to the kitchen had large gaps beneath them. Lights that attract night flying insects were located directly above the external doors. The dumpsters were really trashy. They had nice lids (district-wide) but the lids weren't being used. They were small-capacity dumpsters which I believed should have been replaced by larger ones that are easier to maintain. In the custodial closet "barf-a-way" (a corn meal product used to sop up vomit) was spilled on the floor (I should keep a bag in my car), and mouse poop abounded. When we inspected the concession stand we found an immature Black Widow Spider, poor mop storage (each dirty strand of a mop, lying on the floor is a "gummy bear" treat for roaches, crickets and ants), and an old retail mouse bait station.

P.S. Diskin Elementary was a whole different story — good-looking school, more suburban than inner city. The staff were very easy to work with, but pest-conducive conditions abounded. In the small kitchen (meals were prepared at a central facility elsewhere) "the firm" had the contract – they pre-baited and used perimeter treatment two times a year. They inspected only twice per year! We found six monitors, all containing roaches (American and Oriental), Indian House and Field Crickets and some Dermestids (Hide Beetles that live on dead animal skin). The shelving and serving areas were of good quality, but some of these units needed sealing. Typical of kitchens where parent teacher organizations can store and sell snacks for fund-raisers, we found locked doors and cupboards, and they were very dirty. Locked doors, of course, prohibited proper monitoring and/or sanitation. I suppose someone was worried that custodians might steal some of their stale, pest-infested popcorn. No pest monitors were evident, but lots of mouse poop and clutter was. Cafeteria exit doors exhibited at least half-inch gaps, which would allow mice and almost any insect access — they needed door sweeps! The staff lounge was clean, but with the standard vending area that mice and roaches love. The storage room was clean, but contained many cardboard boxes and harborage (clutter that protects pests from predators and adverse weather conditions). Teachers love to create harborage.

Ed Van Tobel Middle School was very similar to the middle school at the Kyrene School District in Tempe with respect to conducive conditions. Really nice folks, the two vice-principals accompanied us, as did the head custodian and kitchen supervisor. We saw dead sewer roaches in profusion. We did have a report of "punkies" (biting gnats) attacking one classroom. My bet was they were related to rains and new construction next door.

The cafeteria custodial closet had a rotted-out wall with evidence of a German Cockroach infestation (adult female with ootheca – egg cases). In the kitchen, floors and equipment were relatively clean (except for spilled bug juice), but the floor drains were in bad shape. "The firm's" monitors indicated Dermestids, German Cockroaches, Firebrats and spiders. Of course, the traps were unlabeled. Food containers (cans and boxes) were not dated for proper rotation (practicing first-in, first-out offers less time for stored food product pests to infest or reproduce). The teacher's lounge looked very clean at first glance. Teachers were there eating lunch during our inspection, and laughed at our stories of how teachers cause pests. However, when I jumped up on the counter to check out tops of cupboards and found an old mouse nest, they ceased eating. One teacher stopped talking to me at that point. I guess it was my fault.

For the most part, prior to the implementation of this pilot program at PA Diskin Elementary School, Edward Von Tobel Middle School and Rancho High School, the district was applying pesticides inside and at the periphery of school facilities, without monitoring for pests, at the request of untrained personnel and not according to any schedule. Chronic pests such as ants, roaches, crickets and mice were frequently reported. In other words, potentially dangerous pesticides were being applied, yet pest problems persisted. Further, pesticide storage procedures practiced by district personnel were inadequate and the district notification policy for spraying pesticides was outdated. As is common with most school districts throughout the country, the Clark County School District structural pest management program was implemented by the facilities management and food services administrators who used minimally trained, but certified, employees and/or contract personnel. Virtually no communication or cooperation about common pests and pesticide use existed among facilities, food and academic services and the licensed Pest Control Operator or pest control contactor.

At this point we considered the pest and conducive conditions to be challenging but workable. My strategy suggested to work with this particular school district (based on receptive administrative mood, current pest situation and motivated employees) was to give them all a lot of "face time" and nurturing for the first four months of the program. We were in for some real education when it came to people management in a large school bureaucracy.

How the Program Progressed

In general, implementation of IPM in the Clark County School District pilot schools was very slow. The implementation team strongly agreed with Bobby's observation(s) that Clark County School District was not practicing effective or safe pest management in the pilot schools. Bobby Corrigan and I had evaluated those schools for pests, pest conducive conditions and pest management strategies; John and I had audited them for pesticide use and pest management costs. Lyn Hawkins monitored them for pests, produced and distributed monthly newsletters, and a significant percentage of staff (including "the firm's" staff) had been trained one-on-one, in classroom, and/or walk-through style since the program was initiated in the summer.

LESSON 6: Be very aggressive and timely when developing and delivering a picture of pest problems, pesticide use information and pest control costs.

It was critical that John Carter and I be able to paint a picture of Clark County School District's past and current pest management practices. Without that picture it would be difficult to determine how or if the program was working, or provide convincing evidence so district decisionmakers could feel comfortable adopting IPM — information that could make the transition more seamless. I don't think we ever got even close to acquiring all the information we needed. This difficulty is common with many school district partners, but Clark County School District was totally lost, knew it and was lying about it.

Unfortunately, the evidence of pests was increasing at Ranch High School. A major reason for this expected increase was that pest-conducive conditions in the pilot schools had not been addressed. In all fairness to Clark County School District, my team had not communicated all conditions promptly (due to delayed training sessions in one instance). Seems our first training session was scheduled two weeks after September 11, 2001. I was in Washington, D.C. when the planes struck the Twin Towers and Pentagon. There was no way I could get to Las Vegas until mid-October. Nonetheless, two specific reasons pointed to the ongoing need for communication:

1) There was a need for increased communication and cooperation between kitchen/custodial staff and maintenance staff about work needed to prevent pests from entering facilities (holes in walls, foundation cracks, overhanging trees, etc.).
2) An apparent reduction of custodial services staff at Rancho High School.

That said, sanitation levels were improving in the Rancho High School kitchen, and we observed some immediate positive response to our initial staff training from the cafeteria custodian, Mr. Blue.

Blue's case was both exciting and sad. We had scheduled a three-day training session with the district eight weeks earlier, and the Operations' training manager assured me all was ready. Custodial, kitchen and grounds staff from our three pilot schools were to attend our two-hour training sessions for three consecutive days. The training was our standard IPM awareness program for staff:

1) What are the pests you have?
2) Why do you have them?
3) What can you do within the confines of your current job responsibilities?

People who work in schools often feel they have too much on their plate, and we never want to portray our program as adding more to that plate. We held our training sessions at Rancho High School in the cafeteria...where Blue worked.

On our second day of training we did some walk-through training, pointing out the evidence of pest presence and the conducive conditions which either attracted them and/or allowed them to infest an area. Pest-vulnerable areas such as kitchens, teachers' lounges, cafeterias, concession stands, science rooms (where pets and their food are kept) and custodial closets/storage rooms are great places to demonstrate this. I took Blue and about 10 other trainees to Blue's storage room in the cafeteria. I had checked it out earlier and found that the same bag of popcorn, greasy popcorn maker and other junk was still in the very same storage room I had inspected the previous summer! Of course, the trainees were grossed out when I showed them the mice poop, dead roaches and crickets that indicated something besides students was living in that room. But, nobody, including me, chastised Blue because we all knew that these were common conditions throughout the school.

Before our final training session on day three I checked out the room again — sometimes prayers get answered. Blue had sanitized that room! It was one of the most outstanding demonstrations of professional initiative I had encountered in the custodial community. Accordingly, I had the whole class witness the change and asked Blue to explain what he found and who he had had to consult for permission to dump the popcorn. First he mentioned that, after our initial visit, he had also found live roaches in the popcorn and a lot more mice poop, "It was nasty!" he said. As it happened, the popcorn and junk belonged to the coach... which meant Blue had to walk on eggshells to explain the situation. Please know that this took no small amount of courage, as coaches are on the top of the food chain in schools throughout the country. (Indeed, most principals cringe in their presence.) Fortunately, the coach saw the disgusting mess for himself and granted Blue permission to dump it all.

I wish this story had a happy ending. Unfortunately, just as the last group was leaving the storage room, one custodian asked Blue if his nose "could be any browner". What a piece of work this woman was to deride a fellow worker for doing the right thing for his job, himself and school children. And not one co-worker defended Blue. This experience left a bad taste in everyone's mouth, and demonstrated a perfect example of the need for "cultural control". In this case, the custodial community culture at this school was so poorly managed that it felt no professional obligation to confront sanitary conditions that might be harmful to the rest of the school community. In case you missed it, my indictment is of the district /administration. Through its actions (staff cutbacks and using this decrepit environment as a training area, or worse, a dumping ground for administrators), the administration had abandoned Rancho High School in the eyes of the people responsible for ensuring sanitary conditions.

Further, school custodians from Diskin and Von Tobel couldn't attend training. Lyn Hawkins subsequently conducted one-on-one training sessions for them. The county health official and State Lead representative also didn't make it to training. "The firm" sent a representative for just one day. The Clark County School District training specialist and I attempted to schedule this training to ensure maximum attendance and minimum disruption. Attendance and participation from Rancho custodial staff was good, but there were communication problems with Grounds and Kitchen staff that reduced attendance. Attendance would have been better if the administration said, "make it so", but we ourselves also should have been more considerate.

LESSON 7: Be more considerate of the school's staff's availability before scheduling training.

Training for subsequent programs should be conducted at each pilot school. Principals and staff find it difficult to allow "off campus" training. Custodial staff work in two shifts. Current training is available to only one shift. We now recommend that the walk-through sessions be conducted for each shift.

Clark County is a very large school district undergoing almost unbelievable growth and administrative transition. Facility administrators seemed overwhelmed with both, and thus are not particularly attentive to the needs and desires of the implementation team and IPM program implementation. As with most IPM program initiations, these crisis-oriented administrators were having real problems elevating IPM to anything beyond polite (and most were very polite) indifference. This attitude is common, but seemed more pronounced in such a large bureaucracy. Anonymous comments later suggested, "Your program and recommendations would have been better received if the school district had paid for it."

LESSON 8: Get commitment from the highest level of administration before getting in too deep

- Problems with the Clark County School District pursuant to the success of this pilot program were of commitment and communication. The school district could have remedied these problems by developing and distributing to Facilities managers and pilot school principals a signed statement from the superintendent committing the district to the concept of safer, more effective pest management through the successful demonstration of IPM.

LESSON 9: Identify and use a children's environmental health advocate, particularly in large, bureaucratic school districts.

I mentioned this lesson earlier in this book. Change works best when it is voluntary — when a school district perceives the IPM innovation to be relatively advantageous, not too complex and something it can try out and observe. In this case the change agents really are there to provide information and a lot of hand holding. School administrators, as educational professionals, usually have a relatively high opinion of the change agents we work with. However, when a school system is so large or so poorly run that it allows petty bureaucrats to manage adoption of IPM (and they are not willing to put out the necessary effort) political pressure is required. This pressure comes best from the school community itself. As I have mentioned, a determined and informed mother with a babe in arms has a major influence on school boards. Moms can fight the fight better than university or government bug people.

Results (well, sort of) and Recommendations

The State Lead Agency initiated the idea of this program in Nevada, and therefore should be commended for its progressive attitude concerning pollution prevention rather than "command and control" strategies for pesticide users, children's health protection and school fiscal responsibility. Charles Moses shared this strategy with other State Lead Agencies at a Pesticide Regulator Education Program. He even offered the Clark County School District funding opportunities if it would open the appropriate funding accounts, but the district never did.

Sticky trap monitors were sited in significant pest-vulnerable areas in each pilot school. Scheduled pesticide applications were eliminated or only low impact pesticides (no or very low mammalian toxicity) were applied as-needed. One elementary school actually required had no pesticide applications, while another still applied baits for ants. The high school was not using pesticides and exhibited a decrease in pests. However, we expected an increase in pest reports at the high school during the next spring after our pilot program concluded. We expected the increase because conducive conditions in the pilot schools had not been addressed. There was a need for increased communication and cooperation between kitchen/custodial staff and maintenance staff regarding work needed to prevent pests from entering facilities (holes in walls, foundation cracks, overhanging trees, etc.); and an apparent reduction of custodial services staff at Rancho High School contributed to decreased sanitation and morale.

While the pilot schools' staff improved their sanitation and maintenance practices, the implementation team assumed that related practices throughout the district did not change. In all fairness to the district, Clark County School District had outgrown a pest management strategy which probably once worked, and in fact still is practiced by most (though smaller) school districts throughout the country. A reasonable ratio for a full-time, full-service professional pest manager is 1:50 — Pest Management Professionals to schools (six high schools, eight middle schools and 36 elementary schools). This ratio is based on four schools per day, two hours per school (inspection, monitoring, treatment, communication, paperwork and travel), plus additional time for intensive remediation and follow-up communication.

After reviewing our results and discussing the numerous problems and possible solutions for the Clark County programs I developed the following recommendations for the district's assistant superintendent:

Recommendations for the School District's Administration

1. Recognize what a quality pest manager is and what a reasonable workload for that person should be.
2. Standardize the district by having uniform training requirements and joint in-service training for any pest manager.
3. Professionalize the district by expanding staff qualifications and increasing compensation to industry standards.
4. The district should consider combining and internalizing pest management responsibilities, focusing on the school as the unit of operation rather than the program area (food service, grounds, facilities).

5. Review technical recommendations from the implementation team and assist the pilot schools in their understanding of remedial measures for conducive conditions.

6. Document the remediation of conducive conditions by the pilot schools.

7. Develop and implement an aggressive ant management program for Diskin Elementary School with the assistance of Drs. Corrigan and Lame.

8. Concentrate Rancho High School pest management activities in the cafeteria complex (kitchen, dock, cafeteria, storage rooms and teachers lounge) to demonstrate conducive condition remediation and rodent control.

9. Schedule development, release and distribution of three more monthly newsletters (issue topics: ants, roaches and mice/spiders) with the program coordinator, district training specialist and pilot school principals.

By and large, these recommendations were what we had asked the assistant superintendent's administrations to implement the previous year. The less-school-specific recommendations were similar to those we had used with our other programs. Fortunately, with those other school districts, the recommendations were heeded within several months of the initiation of new programs.

At the end of our program with Clark County I met with the district assistant superintendent to convince him that this program could work, but to do so it needed more administrative commitment. Although some school districts throughout the country were beginning to view the implementation of pesticide accountability programs (notification of the school community when pesticides are used and IPM) as the "right thing to do", many just didn't know where to begin. Such a beginning is what we had offered the school district. Although this administrator wanted to say his district was, indeed, "doing the right thing", he expressed interest in expanding the program only on a cost-neutral basis. While I didn't like this message, I understood it. I went to work to figure out how the school district could do this. The following was my final report to the district decisionmakers:

> Two avenues exist through which outside funding could be obtained for Clark County School District: 1) Become a PESP partner and thus become eligible for competitive USEPA grants (normally less than $50,000); and 2) set up an account that allows the State Lead Agency (Chuck Moses at the Nevada

Department of Agriculture) to deposit monies collected from structural pesticide use violations. The current program implementation team is very willing to provide assistance with either of these options.

The concept of cost neutrality for Clark County School District is questionable if one considers that current expenditures are far below those needed to maintain professional pest management standards. Using figures provided by the district and a survey conducted by Chuck Moses, we found Clark County School District was spending an average of $500/school (234 schools in the district at the time). The range of spending varies widely: $466 per middle and high school average (treated monthly) to $60 per elementary school (treated semi-annually) as Food Service expenditures, and a $286 per school average from Operations (your Pest Control Operator's salary plus materials). These figures do not include administrative costs such as those incurred when notifying the school community when pesticide applications are scheduled.

A previous audit at the Kyrene School District in Tempe, Arizona, conducted by John using the same methodology, indicated that schools there (elementary and middle only) were spending approximately $700/year, with administrative costs as high as $300/year. It is our experience that for a typically sized school district, pest management costs average approximately $1,000 per school (pest management personnel, materials and administrative costs).

As with the vast majority of districts in the country, Kyrene did not delineate pest management as a separate line item in overall operations budget. Thus, in the initial analysis it was apparent that the district ascribed a nominal budget for the contractual cost of pest management in 25 schools. Upon further analysis, we determined that the actual cost of pest management (contract + extra pesticide applications + administrative hours) was approximately three times the original estimate. This finding illustrates what our team is finding in all program areas: that traditional pest management is no more cost-effective than a quality IPM program, is less efficient at addressing short- and long-term pest problems/complaints and unnecessarily exposes children and adult inhabitants of the school to pesticides.

Using the broad assumptions that administrative costs would be vastly reduced by adopting a notification policy which

> exempts baits and gels, and virtually eliminating more toxic applications (as demonstrated in all of our pilot programs), and factoring in an economy of scale effect, a large school district could end up spending as little as $700/school per year. That is less than Clark County School District currently spends for combined Food Service/Facilities pest management services in its middle and high schools. Further, Clark County School District appears to have a competent and willing training staff that could reduce costs by internalizing professional pest management.
>
> There is no way your current contracted semi-annual, preventive pesticide treatment can be called IPM, nor is it effective in pest-vulnerable areas. Monthly monitoring/inspection should be the standard. The total $350 (contracted Pest Control Operator plus your Pest Control Operator) spent annually at Clark County School District elementary schools is not only far below the average, but also appears not to be cost effective.

Included with this report was my plan for district-wide expansion by internalizing the pest management responsibilities in one of their five regional districts — focusing on the school as the unit of operation rather than the program area (food service, grounds, facilities); positioning and training a certified pest manager for implementing IPM; and implementing a region-wide IPM education program for teachers, staff and administrators (newsletters and training). Knowing I had already earned a too pushy reputation with some of the assistant superintendent's administrators, I suggested that someone other than me become the plan coordinator.

Clark County School District opted to ignore these recommendations, declined offers to assist with expansion funding, and the superintendent refused to return phone calls. I understand that principals at the pilot elementary schools are still using IPM and have attempted to spread it throughout the district.

LESSON 10: The Monroe IPM Model does not work in poorly managed school districts.

The Clark County School District was just the beginning of my understanding that no matter how hard the IPM implementation team tries, unless the district is both committed and well managed, our program (which is based on communication) will not work. Pest management is people management. You can't manage pests unless people are managed, too. Activists might force the ill-managed district to function. If that does not work, public decisionmakers must enact, fund and enforce laws that will require those already being paid to protect our children to protect them better.

Chapter Ten - Reservations about the Reservation – The Navajo Nation

In early 2001 the USEPA, Office of Pesticide Programs contacted me to see if we could develop a pilot program for IPM in the Bureau of Indiana Affairs (BIA) school facilities on the Navajo Indian Reservation. It seemed that no one had ever looked at what the BIA was doing for pest management in reservation schools. The very dangerous pathogen Hantavirus, which is transmitted by the deer mouse, stimulated some interest in how we might prevent this type of problem in reservation schools. The USEPA had presented the results of our programs in Arizona to the BIA environmental folks and got an enthusiastic response. I guess it looked like a workable project, and they asked me to head out to Crown Point, New Mexico, (ground zero for the last Hantavirus epidemic) and see if it could be done.

Now, many entomologists have traveled the world looking at bugs, but I am not one of them. I just never got around to it. The only time I was asked to go to an exotic place I declined. Of course, that was Vietnam in 1971. However, I believe that many of us natural science types fantasize ourselves as khaki-clad explorers in exotic places. Growing up partially in the Southwest gave me some exposure to Native Americans and, of course, I viewed their culture as exotic compared to mine. Further, I had worked with many of the tribes both at Extension, and even more when I was with the Arizona Department of Environmental Quality where one of my job responsibilities was to be tribal liaison to the 25 tribes in the state.

I knew that Indian reservations were way under-funded in the area of environmental protection. And, believe it or not, while many of our Native

Americans are acutely aware of their ties to nature (Mother Earth), they are not as in touch with the environmental consequences of "modern living" in a technical sense. I believe this is because it has been convenient for our government, some industries and certain unscrupulous tribal leaders (yes, all cultures have them) to suppress environmental awareness and regulation. That allows tribes and their partners (e.g., uranium mining, clear cutting forests, hazardous/radioactive waste storage and disposal to indulge environmentally risky behavior and sale tactics that result in overuse of pesticides — particularly herbicides). In my Environmental Management class at Indiana University I address these types of situations under the heading of "environmental justice". This issue is sometimes called "environmental racism", whereby a disenfranchised community is exposed to unequal distribution of environmental risk (O'Leary, 1999).

Except for a few very interesting attitudes regarding what we consider pests, folks in Indian Country feel about and deal with pests the same way the rest of America does. They don't want to live with them and are willing to do what they have to in order to compete with them. Let's be clear here. They watch the same commercials that we do, and some use the hell out of pesticides just as so many other Americans do. Anyway, I sat in on a conference call with the feds in D.C., the BIA's Eastern Navajo Agency school facilities people in Crown Point and the Navajo EPA pesticide regulators. I got an idea of what was going on there and who I would be working with, and shortly after I made my way out to "the Rez".

BIA has five "agencies" on the Navajo Indian Reservation/Navajo Nation (some in Arizona and some in New Mexico) which is the largest reservation in the continental United States. My assessment began at the Eastern Navajo Agency Facility Offices in Crown Point, New Mexico, about 40 miles from Gallup. I met with a work group that consisted of members of the Tribe (Navajo EPA), BIA facility managers and the contracted pest control operator. Three of the 18 schools managed by the BIA had been selected for this program initiation — Crown Point Community School, Lake Valley School and Mariano Lake School. At this meeting, we discussed the conditions (which, by now, we had outlined in our MOU) necessary to implement a successful program. In particular, we outlined the need to have a committed school administration, an on-site program manager, the opportunity to conduct an audit (documenting current pest problems, pesticide use and cost of pest management), and the training of facility personnel (regarding how to prevent pest infestations, recognize pest contusive conditions and how to remediate those conditions). I found attendees at this meeting to be very receptive, particularly the facilities manager, Bob Villarreal, and his Environmental Specialist (a position unique to the Eastern Navajo Agency) Chad Bourgoin.

While the Navajo EPA folks were very interested in implementing IPM, I noticed they were not overly willing to work with the BIA. This animosity goes back to the late 1800s and stems from the sovereign status of the tribe and its relationship with its U.S. government "overseers" – the BIA. Quite naturally, the tribes resent the authority that BIA commands on the reservation. Conversely, BIA personnel have mandates to follow, and believe their input is needed to assure standards for education, health, etc. This is an old and ongoing mess over which the Department of the Interior (where the BIA is administratively located) and tribes throughout the U.S. are deadlocked— particularly as it pertains to Indian "trust" monies. I learned there were "BIA Schools" and "Tribal Schools", and was beginning to realize I would not be able to work with both in the initial stages of implementation.

Crown Point Community School, Lake Valley School, and Mariano Lake School all were BIA schools, while Crown Point was actually in the town of Crown Point. Lake Valley and Mariano Lake are located in more traditional villages. Most BIA schools have dormitories where students live during the school week. This would become a particularly challenging aspect to our project with when it came to managing pests. Also, it was a real learning experience with regard to communicating with a particular audience. Being aware of the big Indian School in Phoenix, I had always heard that Navajos, Hopi, Apache, Pima and other tribal children were forced out of their homes and villages and made to live in schools controlled by the government so they could learn the ways of the white man. These days the dormitory schools are located in or near villages of the student population and are very culturally oriented with regard to language, traditions, etc.

I was surprised that the schools and dorms were receptive to being developed as models. BIA personnel had warned me that these were "rough places" when it came to pest-conducive conditions. However, I found the facilities to be in good condition regarding both building repair and sanitation. After some of the schools I had seen in our previous pilot programs (particularly Rancho High School in Las Vegas) it would have been hard to call these schools "rough places". I attributed the better-than-expected conditions to above-average facility management and to the fact that the Indian Health Service inspected the facilities (regarding sanitation) more frequently than we did in non-Tribal public schools.

Evidently, these inspectors were very concerned about disease transmission. Hantavirus is very scary stuff. In the early 1990s dozens of people were killed by this rodent-borne disease (in the urine and feces of the deer mouse). Every year several more residents of the area contract the disease. Some die. Most now survive, but sometimes are permanently disabled. Thus, the community is acutely aware of the disease as it is related to sanitation and rodent exclusion necessary for prevention. From our point of view, this awareness would aid in implementing additional cultural controls for pests other than mice. It is interesting that this area of the country also produces one or two cases of plague (as in The Black Plague) every year. Plague is a flea-borne disease associated with rodents. No matter whom your audience, you can always get immediate attention when you mention plague.

Rodent prevention practices in the schools for exclusion and chemical baiting were inadequate. Entryways for deer mice were evident in all the schools. Many of the external doorways had ground-level gaps that allowed entry to mice. If you can fit a pencil beneath any door or crack in the foundation, a mouse can squeeze through (Corrigan, 2001). Of greatest concern were portable classrooms built above ground. Structural openings for pipes, electrical conduit, etc., were unsealed and conducive to pest entry. Because of the threat of disease transmission, snap traps for deer mice are not used in reservation schools. Therefore, control of mice that might enter the school facility was limited to poison baits. On the good side, the pest control contractor was not using the pelleted baits that can be translocated by mice, instead utilizing the larger biscuit type bait. Unfortunately, these baits had been improperly distributed and were not containerized. They were not as effective as they should have been and also presented a potential danger to smaller children in the schools. Pretty green biscuits can be tempting to hungry five- and six–year-olds.

Following discussion with the work group and a cursory inspection of the pilot schools/dorms, I found pest pressures to be low. Flying insects and spiders (bees, wasps, and house flies) were not a problem in terms of presence or tolerance, and roaches were non-existent. This region has a very dry climate and is at a high altitude that makes it tough on traditional structural pests. I did find one of the very large (six to 10 inches long) centipedes common to the region and heard of the very occasional scorpion. Harvester Ants and what residents called Sugar Ants were present and considered to be pests. Sugar Ants entered facilities via cracks and crevices. Harvester Ants were found only outside the buildings. Harvester Ants or Pogos (a shortened scientific name – from genus *Pogonomyrmex*) are very common in the desert Southwest. A large ant, they almost never sting, but they can. Years ago when I was working on Rangeland Caterpillars in Northeastern New Mexico I got one up my

142

pants, and when she finally decided to sting me, I was driving down the freeway. In abject pain, I pulled over, dropped my pants and scraped her off. My leg cramped for the rest of the day, and my always-compassionate colleagues questioned whether any kind-hearted motorists had offered to stop and help me with my pants.

Of real interest to us entomologist types were the more-than-occasional head lice and bedbug infestations. When visiting Fort Wingate High School I did get to visit a dorm room that had recently been treated for a massive infestation of bedbugs. I actually was able to locate live specimens without much trouble — after the insecticide treatments! This is really neat stuff in that bedbugs were considered a common pre-WWII pest, but became fairly rare with the widespread use of DDT and other pesticides in homes and hotels. I had never seen a live specimen until that visit to Fort Wingate. Evidently, the environment in the high deserts of New Mexico is great for bedbugs. That, with the decreased use of certain pesticides, has allowed a resurgence of these blood suckers in many places in the state. In fact, hotels throughout the country are beginning to experience an inkling of the bedbug problems that were so common before the 1950s. Vertebrate pests other than rodents did not seem to be much of a problem among the Navajo schools. We did have some ravens visiting the dumpsters outside the kitchen areas. We also had a litter of puppies living in one of the dumpsters — wild dogs are common on the Rez. Some facility maintenance men did remove several rattlesnakes from under a portable school room while I was visiting. Folks weren't too excited. Navajos will not kill snakes, and you commonly find them around buildings.

Like most Pest Control Operators, the BIA contractor was practicing as a traditional exterminator (and is the head of this family business) relying on chemical pesticide control for both prevention and remediation. However, unlike many pest control contractors, he seemed totally accepting of the IPM concept and of morphing into a diagnostician/educator. As a member of the Tribe and having a multi-decade professional relationship with the school district, he was into practicing pest management the best way possible. (Note that while his firm had practiced on the Reservation for years, he had just recently contracted for the three pilot schools we would be working in.) It was my understanding that BIA personnel had been conducting pest control prior to his contract, and that they were into the nuclear (as in let's "nuke 'em") mode of application.

According to the exterminator and the school facilities manager, all bugs were being treated at least a bi-monthly with a scheduled application of a synthetic pyrethroid insecticide. I witnessed such a treatment by one of the contractor's technicians. He used approximately one gallon of solution per facility building. The insecticide was haphazardly applied to the baseboards and directly on ant mounds. In general, there was no indication that pesticides were needed for any of the standard pests we normally encountered. Thus, here was our first opportunity to demonstrate drastic pesticide use reduction. I also noted that when pesticides were indicated for very limited situations, they were not effectively used. Mattresses, walls and baseboards were treated for the specific bedbug infestation I witnessed. However, this treatment did not include any flushing agents that would force the reclusive bloodsuckers from cracks and crevices on or around the beds, or the folds of the bedding, to expose them to the pesticide. Nor were there scheduled follow-up treatments which would break the lifecycle of this pest. Timing and coverage are everything when it comes to the effective use of pesticides. Like antibiotics, if you don't use them correctly, they can do more harm than good. No monitoring traps were being used for any pests. The pest control contractor made no attempt to educate facility managers about pest prevention. Clearly, there was plenty of room for improvement in terms of sophistication and unnecessary pesticide use.

This contractor committed to upgrade his firm's methods to IPM, and I felt he would be great to work with. His firm consisted of him, his son and nephew. The latter two were both unlicensed technicians (typical in the business). The head guy told me that the last time he saw an inspector from the New Mexico Department of Agriculture (which inspects and tests licensed Pest Control Operators) was years ago. We wanted to get them to some organized training for structural IPM — probably at Dawn's workshop in Phoenix. Most important, they did attend our assessment and training in Crown Point and Lake Valley and seemed to be very motivated, which was different than our experience with other programs. The team hoped to give them a lot of face time on their monthly visits.

The Team

Not surprisingly, when I contacted Bobby Corrigan, Jerry Jochim, Mike Lindsey, Dawn Gouge and Carl Martin to team with me on this project, they all jumped at the chance. Mike, Carl and I had worked on reservations before. In fact, Carl (who had become a major risk-taker with Arizona's Structural Pest Control Board) had spent two years on the Rez as a Mormon Missionary and spoke fluent Navajo. Bobby and Dawn had not spent any appreciable time on an Indian reservation. Since they're from other countries (England and New York City), Dawn and Bobby couldn't wait to put on headdresses and smoke peace-pipes. I should also mention that Bobby and Dawn were keenly interested in Hantavirus management. Hell, so was I! We talked Carl Olson (who I believe is the best insect identification man in the Southwest) into joining us, after very minor arm twisting. So it wasn't hard to coordinate everyone for our initial assessments and trainings. After working together for several years, we knew the drill.

We looked forward to our six-hour drives from Phoenix to our designated HQ, the El Rancho Hotel in Gallup. Normally, we would stop for one break in the desert and one in the mountains north of Strawberry, Arizona, to stretch our legs and look under rocks and logs for different arthropods. Honing our assessment skills by finding and identifying all manner of bugs is sport to folks like us. Carl Olson and Mike normally did some fine teaching while Jerry and Carl Martin suffered our childish delight in playing with bugs. After several years together we were really improving and integrating our skills. This all sounds like fun (and is), but it is also critical team development: A <u>good</u> manager recognizes when a team approach is needed, who should make up that team and how to choose the team members. Then that <u>good</u> manager will develop the team through briefings, debriefings, skill sharing and social interaction: Best folks + best communication = the best result. Not only will that team produce a quality program with the best possible results, but each team member also will become his/her own regional team leader. It's a snowball effect. Too bad that many Extension entomologists are rarely trained to be <u>good</u> managers.

The local BIA team decided Chad Bourgoin would be our on-site IPM coordinator. Chad had a background in environmental management, was highly intelligent and motivated. We were very concerned he was not a professional pest manager, but were pretty confident he was a quick learner. The fact is, he was the only person on-site who could do the job. It would turn out to be a problem, but one we were able to overcome. Fortunately, Chad was able to attend our staff training and mid-term evaluation in Las Vegas so he could get a feel for how we conduct these types of programs. It was very good for him in terms of program initiation, pest identification and monitoring procedures. It also allowed him to see how screwed up the Clark County School District was, compared to his own school facilities. I had hoped he could stimulate BIA education facilities management on other Indian reservations to develop the environmental specialist position. Chad's boss, Bob Villarreal, was an ex-Air Force, ex-DOD facility manager with lots of experience, and he liked what we were bringing him. He was the local boss and could make things happen. For all intents and purposes this was our school district administration, and, per our standard MOU, it looked like we had our required commitment from BIA and the Tribe to provide records, staff and take our recommended actions. The person who was really driving the BIA commitment was an environmental scientist with the BIA out of D.C. – Debbie McBride. She was a Navajo woman who really knew her culture first-hand. She had discovered that BIA really wanted to implement IPM. We were hopeful she could provide political clout to make this happen, and expand.

We had three regulators from the Navajo EPA Pesticide Unit in Window Rock. It was my understanding that they were funded by and reported to EPA region 9 — much like a State Lead Agency. The Navajo EPA folks would be partners, but mostly observers, in anticipation of the expansion of the program. The Tribal/USEPA relationship was problematic. EPA Region 9 was concerned that the Navajo pesticide staff were overloaded with current pesticide regulatory responsibilities, and it didn't want them to take on much more. In some ways, this relationship was much like the relationship between USEPA Regions and most states (command and control). However, the relationship was more politically sensitive because of the sovereign status of tribes. The BIA had reasonably good control over how its schools were managed, and was concerned that the tribal Grant Schools would be harder to use as pilot schools. The Tribal folks felt a bit left out. I hoped we could develop a timeline in which we could officially bring the Grant Schools on board.

How the program progressed

As with all of our pilots, this one got off to a slow start. Working with the feds is always slow. Combine that slowness with an institution that operates in the most isolated parts of our country, where time takes on a different meaning, very strange politics and excessive travel time. I started wishing I was working with the BIA in Ohio. Of course, our ancestors made sure there were no reservations in Ohio. Anyway, between getting the local folks in Crown Point to organize our first training and formal assessments, the travel time to get to the Rez, and working around the terrorists 9/11 attack travel restrictions, we didn't get our training completed until the following spring. However, we did convince Chad to suspend pesticide use (other than rodent baits) in all the pilot schools, based on my initial assessment. Like I said, there just wasn't any need to be using pesticides when no situation indicated that pesticides would be helpful. As is typical in new programs, we had some communication problems. One allowed Mariano Lake to be treated for lice just prior to our first team visit— what a waste. However, this specific incident did educate my team about the significance of "bugs" in the Navajo culture, and the pervasiveness of Madison Avenue's high pressure sales messages.

We arrived for a briefing with Chad and his handlers at the BIA facilities building in Crown Point, the morning of our first formal assessments and staff training sessions at the pilot schools. During the briefing Chad mentioned that a classroom had been sprayed for lice. Because he had attended our Las Vegas trainings, he knew there was no such thing as a legitimate area application of pesticides for lice, and he also knew I would get damn' upset about it. In his laid-back way he related what we had heard so many times before: A teacher discovered that one of her students had head lice and demanded that the contractor spray her classroom. Because the teacher, custodian and principal thought spraying would rid everyone of lice, and the exterminator didn't know any better (or worse, did know better), everyone thought it was okay. Of course this is a waste of money and dangerous to the children, but the industry promotes pesticides as a cure for any bugs, and these folks bought it.

The very interesting thing here is that traditional Navajos don't hate bugs. Debbie explained that while Navajos don't want lice, there is no stigma regarding the presence of this human ecto-parasite. In fact, the Navajo regard head lice as "the bug which brings the people together". Indeed, "preening" each other for lice was an important social function in most cultures throughout the world. Now our "civilized cultures" have opted to apply poison to our scalps. Unfortunately, the industry is willing to apply poison to our environment to make us believe we have no problem with lice, and our teachers are told that no lice should be in their schools. Broadcast use of pesticides must be the answer!

The Navajo also will not step on or squash spiders. They believe spiders are symbolic of "Spider Woman" who taught them the life skill of weaving. Even so, they don't want spiders in their schools or living quarters. Frustrating is that, while the traditional Navajo will not mechanically kill a spider, there seems to be a disconnect in this logic in that it's okay to spray them. In that case, they "go away". Is this a story of aboriginal thinking? I don't think so. What about my children's willingness to eat steak, wrapped in cellophane purchased from a store, but not eat meat from an animal that I slaughtered and butchered myself? Haven't they disconnected the wrapped meat from the flesh of a doe-eyed animal? What caused this disconnect? Our need for convenience? Who caused this? Madison Avenue and its ability to make us believe that meat comes from supermarkets, and pesticides can just make bugs disappear. This is why we try to educate the school community, so that it can relearn the cause-and-effect relationship between community actions and the presence of pests.

Throughout 2002, Bobby, Jerry, Mike and I conducted five one-on-one training sessions for the pest control contractor, kitchen and custodial supervisors at the pilot schools. Training dealt with identification of pests and pest-conducive situations. Working with the contractor became increasingly more difficult. While he was supportive of IPM he was unwilling to commit to training for himself and his staff so they could really implement IPM as diagnosticians/educators. The contractor was a good man, but he didn't believe that the community (school or otherwise) really wanted IPM. Further, he felt that his business did not need to go in this direction. When Chad made it a contractual obligation that the contractor use only IPM, this guy decided he had enough traditional exterminator customers to support his business, and he was probably right. In the latter part of this pilot he declined to cooperate with our offers of training or recommendations. This actually worked out well because it forced Chad to work with his superiors to require the two BIA Pest Control Operators to take on the Eastern Navajo Agency schools and begin practicing IPM. As it turned out, these guys couldn't wait to learn more and professionalize. They even drove down to Phoenix to attend one of Dawn's workshops on urban IPM.

Herb Holgate from Navajo EPA attended one of our training sessions. Herb really wanted us to work with the schools run by the Tribe. During this session he grabbed Mike and told him they were "going for a ride". They disappeared for about two hours. It turns out he wanted to let someone on our team know that the program should be expanded to the tribal schools. So what he did was invite Mike, who was the eldest member of our team, to ride out to some centuries-old ruins and discuss the situation. He shared his feelings, in a very cultural environment, with our "elder". This was a communication strategy we had to respect. Even if we knew Mike was just a big kid, he was perceived as a decisionmaker. We had to be more inclusive of the "elders" in the Navajo community. Unfortunately, neither the BIA nor the USEPA took this intercultural approach to communication seriously. In addition, the leader of the Navajo EPA Pesticide Program did not want to communicate with us. To-date, we have not been able to integrate IPM into the tribal schools, but because we had great folks (like Bob King at the Lake Valley School and our own Carl Martin) who helped us understand our audience. we did learn some important lessons in intercultural communication.

We did use some of those lessons learned when we presented the next two training programs for pilot school administrators, teachers, custodial and food service staff. Mostly it was a matter of learning how to show more respect and listen to this particular audience. No doubt this is something we should apply to any audience. Most people are alike. They want to feel like what they do is important, that you respect them, and that you are not too full of your own importance. This we did well, as the team members enjoyed making fun of each other. The Navajo have a great sense of humor and found it particularly hilarious when Bobby, wearing his New York Yankees cap, would put on the accent and tell them how New Yorkers manage pests. This degree of intimacy allows us to discuss really sensitive subjects about personal hygiene, and dormitory, kitchen and classroom conducive conditions with any audience. In these cases we needed always to remember that we were talking about someone's job performance and possibly their cultural values.

The only serious pests in these schools were directly related to conducive conditions. Sanitation was good and maintenance staff were "tightening up" the buildings to prevent deer mice from entering buildings. Once identified correctly, the ant problems just disappeared. Pest identification is always important, but it's critical with ants. Thanks to our Arizona entomologists, the Sugar Ant became the harmless Pyramid Ant, and with some education about conducive conditions, it became a non-pest (Gouge, et. al., 2004). However, thanks to the presence of dorms in the schools, bed bugs were still a problem.

Bed bugs usually were brought into the dorms by just one or two individuals when returning from home with infested bedding or clothes. The bed bugs would feed at night, then hide and reproduce in the cracks of the beds or seams of the mattresses. On one of our drives back to Phoenix the team came up with a plan to reduce bed bugs and the pesticides that were being used against them. First, we suggested a bed bug education plan for the dorm staff, students and their parents to provide them with the reasons why bed bugs were getting into the dorms, and how to prevent them from entering. Basically we wanted to make sure the returning students did not bring any hitchhiking bed bugs from home into the dorms. This would be done by inspecting and laundering incoming bedding. We suggested that the BIA replace wooden bunk-beds in the dorms with ones of different construction and purchase "seamless" mattresses. Apparently the principals of these schools felt that the old army beds looked too institutional, so they purchased wooden beds more homey in appearance. Unfortunately the wooden bed construction included plenty of cracks and crevasses for bed bug harborage. The old army beds had more seamless construction. I don't know if this was by design, but I think the original military specifications for beds might just have included bed bug prevention. They probably haven't changed since WWI when there were lots of bed bugs available for troop quarter infestation. We left it up to Chad to procure beds that prevented harborage but also weren't too institutional in appearance. This falls under the heading of cultural control. We also felt we should explore the idea of using heat to kill the hidden pests. That could be done either by moving the beds into the summer sun once a year or actually increasing the temperature inside the dorms with a special heating device. Lastly we suggested that chemical pesticides be used more effectively (very surgical applications and with a flushing agent) and noted they could be augmented with diatomaceous earth. Diatomaceous earth is abrasive to the cuticle (skin) of insects, causes their bodily fluids to leak out and desiccates them in the process. That's mechanical control. Thus, we developed an IPM program with cultural, mechanical and chemical controls, all based on an educational approach. The start of this special IPM approach for bed bugs had just begun toward the end of our pilot and probably will take years to fully implement.

It takes time for any of our programs to fully be implemented. IPM is a process, not a miracle. In every Monroe IPM Model program we have developed, though pesticides and pests have been drastically reduced, we have yet to get all the teachers and custodians to become partners in the IPM program, even years after the beginning of our program. Why? It is all about changing behavior! I can't think of anything more difficult or time-consuming. The only thing one can do without fear of contradiction is demonstrate success — prove it. For the Navajo pilot schools we demonstrated immediate success by proving drastic reduction in pesticide use, and through the obvious special attention paid to the schools by the BIA facilities staff. Feds are a pain to deal with in some areas, but when it comes to procurement and contracts, once the decision has been authorized by the right folks, things can happen. This was a special lesson for dealing with this type of school system.

Toward the end of the pilot program we recommended that the Eastern Navajo Agency:

- Develop a job description recognizing what a professional pest manager is and what a reasonable workload for that position should be;
- standardize BIA and Tribal pest management professional training requirements and provide joint in-service training for any pest manager;
- "professionalize" by increasing qualifications and compensation to industry standards, and consider combining and internalizing

pest management responsibilities, focusing on the school as the unit of operation rather than the program area (food service, grounds, facilities); and

- develop a pesticide notification policy for all schools.

I also offered the following recommendations to the agency decisionmakers in Washington, D.C.:

1. USEPA and the BIA develop common goals and priorities for the expansion of IPM in Native American schools.
2. Pilot programs be demonstrated on receptive reservations (Navajo, Hopi, Southern Pueblo and Gila River Pima have indicated interest) as models for national expansion.
3. USEPA and BIA develop an MOU for implementing IPM in Native American schools.
4. The USEPA fund a Center for IPM in Schools in USEPA Region 9 to provide technical assistance for the expansion of this Tribal program nationwide, and capitalize on this model of IPM Indian Reservations school districts throughout the Southwest.

Results

After one year in the program we estimated there had been a 95% reduction of pesticide applications in the pilot schools — without additional pest occurrence or cost. Bed bugs did infest the Crown Point dorm midway through the pilot and we had to authorize a very limited application of pesticide until we could implement alternate controls. Agency-wide expansion was implemented by the end of 2002. Because the BIA Eastern Navajo Agency had internalized pest management, we anticipated that all 68 BIA schools (more than 14,000 children) on the Navajo, Southern Pueblo and Hopi Reservations would be able to implement IPM within the next few years.

Perhaps the best way to suggest the program was succeeding is via a recent quote from Chad Bourgoin, "The two PCOs are really getting into the game. Still have not used any pesticide on Eastern Navajo, and we are at 100% implementation. All schools have incorporated the IPM program into a green cleaning program, where the PCO and custodians work to solve issues related to conducive areas" (Bourgoin, Personal Conversation, 2003).

Epilogue

Unfortunately, the BIA has yet to designate more environmental specialists like Chad at school facilities on other reservations. To-date, the Navajo EPA has not implemented IPM in its tribal schools, but other tribes around the country have asked me to send materials so they can implement their own programs. I have been fortunate to be asked to deliver presentations at a number of national tribal environmental meetings. I am still harassing the USEPA and BIA to develop some common goals, priorities and an MOU so they can work together to expand IPM to all Native American schools. Not surprisingly, both agencies won't make that commitment. In fact, they hardly speak to each other. Too bad the current administration in Washington, D.C., seemed almost to benefit from this lack of communication. What about our children?

Within two years the administrative folks with the BIA allowed this success to slip through their hands. They just did not follow up, and never replaced Chad when he left for greener pastures. Even worse, they and their counterparts at the EPA came off as not keeping their word to the school communities on the Navajo Reservation. Both agencies talked as though they would continue funding the maintenance and expansion of IPM with these communities, and they just let it slide. Nothing was done and they came off as promise breakers. Hasn't the Native American community had enough of this already? Of course, that doesn't let that community's leaders off the hook for not "just doing the right thing," regardless of how entities in D.C. held up funding — where there's a will there is a way. The last I heard, the pest management approach on this Rez had reverted to extermination. What a shame.

On a much more positive note, at this point Dawn Gouge and Carl Martin had completely adopted the Monroe IPM Model and began using it in their training sessions. As partners they have used the model in workshops for southwestern Indian Tribes through the Arizona Intertribal Council in Phoenix. Dawn has a very successful program with the Gila River Indian Reservation (once known as the Pima) south of Phoenix and I worked with the Hopi tribal schools. Not bad for an Englishwoman! No doubt, this pilot allowed us to reduce pest problems and the unnecessary exposure of Native American children to pesticides as long as the commitment was there. Even though we all felt the loss of watching our program die on the vine, I promise you we got paid back big time in terms of satisfaction, lessons in big government and intercultural communication, and we got to play explorers in an exotic location.

PART IV:
Tools

Chapter Eleven – The Process for Success - "IPM is a process, not a miracle"

Over our Integrated Pest Management model's years of development I have received many requests from change agents throughout the country for a description of the process one needs to implement what is now called the Monroe IPM Model. With the help of USEPA and the National Foundation for IPM Education, I brought together implementers I had worked with to describe the process we used in persuading school communities to adopt IPM. About 15 of us spent several days together agreeing on this process, its impact on the IPM community, how it should be improved and how to name the model.

In preparation for this "model evaluation meeting" I outlined the steps we used to implement the IPM model. Our group of implementers worked hard to critique each step and recommend improvements. Did we use each step in each program that we had implemented in the previous six years *exactly* the way it should have been used? No, but in the steps listed below we suggest the most effective way and reason to use each step. I can say that before I start any new pilot programs I now review these steps for myself and with my team. They work! When one includes other school districts throughout the country that have consciously incorporated substantial parts of this model into their implementation of IPM, we know that more than a million children have benefited from reduced pest and pesticide exposure.

As discussed in Chapter Five, the successful implementation of any public program requires that three basic questions must be asked and answered: What action must be taken? Who will take that action? And do they have the resources to take the action? (Starling, 1985) The Monroe IPM Model combines the process for answering these simple questions with the Roger's Innovation-Decision process. Below are the 22 steps I believe a good manager should utilize to assure the best chance of adopting a successful school IPM program:

1. Agree: The first thing the IPM model program manager must do is agree with the funding agency on the goals of the model and what resources will be needed. Why do they want you to conduct this program, and what do they want to get out of it? Conversely, what do you want? I hate to say it, but this is negotiation, and you don't stand a chance of getting what you want if you don't know what you want.

For the most part, I have worked with the USEPA, Office of Pesticide Programs, to fund the implementation of this model. They pretty much knew what I wanted to do — to expand the IPM innovation — and how I intended to accomplish this goal. By demonstrating real IPM to a school community, that school community can incorporate it into the school management, and be able to expand IPM to other school communities in the region. It is my experience that the USEPA has these same goals, maybe for more political reasons, but it does see it as part of its general mission, specifically under the mandate of the Federal, Insecticide, Fungicide, Rodenticide Act (FIFRA). I will not accept funding from anyone who does not agree with my definition of IPM and who will not commit to our goals of implementing IPM. However, I am willing to compromise on the goals of expansion, program timing and media exposure. These folks are my partners and I treat them as such. I also expect to be treated as a partner, not as merely a contractor.

The Monroe IPM Model costs the funding agency about $40,000 to implement in an average-size school district. This includes assessments by Professional Pest Managers, administrative overhead (paperwork), recommendations, publicity, travel and on-site inspections by the implementation team. Money is hard to come by for school IPM, and I resent any wasted dollar. This attitude fits pretty well with the requirements for seeking a grant from a government agency. I am not as good when it comes to quarterly reports. However, the Government Performance and Report Act does require this paperwork. I do it, but then I also expect to be able to present the results of our models to others around the country. I believe that government reports left on the shelf are a waste of taxpayer monies.

2. Scout: I always work with the funding agency to strategically plan where the proposed program will have the most chance of success and impact for area-wide expansion. We need the most bang for our bucks. Are the facilities and grounds of the district well managed? Is this a progressive school district that has demonstrated a commitment to other innovative practices and partnerships, either with its facilities or academic excellence? Do the decisionmakers in the district interact with their peers in other districts? Are they leaders? These are questions that should be considered before you and your funding partner invest money, time and reputation.

While it is nice to choose a run-down, pest-infested school district as representative of how the government wants to help out disenfranchised populations, some school districts are run-down and pest-infested for reasons that are incompatible with demonstrating IPM. If a school district cannot manage the behavior of the school community, either because of funding or competence, then positively affecting the sanitation, maintenance and security functions of the district to "do what you are doing now, just think bugs" could be very costly or fail. It is not a matter of old school buildings that have pests; it is how those schools are managed. IPM is a management system and the most cost-effective way to demonstrate the IPM innovation is in a system that is currently well-managed in terms of its sanitation, maintenance and security.

3. Contact: Once you have an idea which school district will offer the most potential for pilot program success and possible regional expansion, you need to establish relationships with interested change agents who reside in the target area (e.g., entomologists, regulatory personal, and children's health activists) and with the representative public school district and the Model implementation team.

Recruiting an Extension Specialist and an On-site IPM coordinator, is not something I do via the Internet. I use my personal and professional network of friends and colleagues who might know someone and/or work in the target area that the funding agency and I have agreed will offer the most potential. Occasionally, the funding agency will have a local contact for me, but often I make my own contacts with the Extension or regulatory folks in the area through networking. It is my experience that without some type of "entry" it is difficult to get these folks to listen to you, let alone work with you. Entries that work best are actually knowing the players, knowing someone else who knows them, and/or mentioning money. I reach as high up as possible — agency directors, department chairs, etc. That way, when or if they have to put you in touch with the person most closely connected to school IPM, that person will know the boss wants something to happen.

School contacts are a little bit more difficult, and I often rely on Extension or regulatory staff to connect me with a school administrator. However, you might be surprised at how many folks you already know who are part of the public education system. Bob King, assistant principal at Lake Valley School on the Rez, turned out to be the brother-in-law of my best friend in Phoenix. So not only did Bob end up being a great help to me during implementation of the Navajo program, but we also got to make fun of our mutual friend behind his back. I have cold-called some school administrators, and usually have been successful obtaining an appointment to discuss the Monroe IPM Model, I usually try the superintendent's office first and always mention my university affiliation and the agency I am working with. Except for the folks in Las Vegas, I have always been treated well. In all cases I bring examples of past programs and newspaper clippings with me. Dr. Tim Gibb at Purdue calls me the schmoozer.

4. Verbal commitment: Since it is a major waste of time to work with a school district that is not really committed, I am fairly assertive from the onset. I insist on communicating with the highest ranking school official (preferably the superintendent) to persuade him/her to say to subordinates and the school community, "I need to try IPM in my schools". This step is obviously different than mere contact because it implies action. I usually walk away if they can't introduce me to the person who has authority to make decisions about pest management in and around the school facilities. It is one thing for school officials to politely listen, and another for them to feel the need to commit resources...and I work very hard to impress them with this fact. They don't want to waste their time either. At this point I make sure they understand how they could benefit or lose when taking on a pilot program. Do I feel like I am wearing a white belt and white shoes while I am selling this used car? No, but I sometimes wonder if I'll be able to deliver the goods

5. Cooperate: Once I am introduced to someone who has appropriate understanding of how facilities are managed (sanitation, maintenance, grounds, etc.) we can begin to cooperatively design a pilot program for the school district. When decisionmakers understand what the Monroe IPM Model is, they can designate schools that will best serve as pilots, based not only on pest pressures, but also on which school principals might be most receptive. They can assist in scheduling and facilitating training programs that are critical for our program, but they also have the authority to divert their staff from their normal duties. By having decisionmakers cooperatively tailor the model to their school district, they begin to own it.

Sweeten the pot: There is risk for both the school district and the funding agency with these pilots, in areas such as time, reputation and money. One way I try to mitigate the risk of adoption is by providing resources. Resources typically take the forms of:

1) Personnel (nationally recognized trainers and assessors with experience at successfully implementing IPM in schools in other states);
2) educational and implementation information and materials;
3) monitoring stations and technical materials; and
4) recognition (awards, publicity, etc.).

Most important: District decisionmakers must be made aware that their political risks are small (they are using a proven program to "do the right thing" for their community), that their actual costs are negligible because this is an externally funded program, and that we are willing and able to do almost all the work.

7. Obtain an MOU (Appendix D): This is a critical step. Obtaining a memorandum of understanding among the school, local change agents (Extension and regulatory), the on-site IPM coordinator and the Implementation Team is not legally binding, but it ethically forces compliance. While I encourage inclusion of the pest control contractor in discussions for this step, I usually do not require the contractor's signature since that person is an "employee" of designated district decisionmakers (usually the facilities manager or assistant superintendent) who are putting their name on the dotted line.

I spell out everything I need to assess the pilot schools, the resources (personnel, time and facilities) I need for training, the historical records we need regarding pest management, the authority to prohibit pesticide applications unless we agree and the possibility of publicizing the program upon successful implementation. In turn, I let all program participants know the resources we will provide, how often and when. I expect everyone to sign the MOU and use it if folks are not holding up their end of the agreement.

8. Assessment/Audit of the School District (Appendix C): This step consists of two parts: 1) The technical assessment of pests, pest-conducive conditions and pest management; and 2) the management assessment of historical and current costs of policies dealing with pest management. This is where the implementation team splits up and goes into the pilot schools. They complete forms for each of the physical and managerial parameters I have listed. This assessment or data is critical as baseline information for program evaluation and also to develop preventive or remedial recommendations for program implementation. The report goes to all members of the implementation team and then to the school district. When the report does get to the designated decisionmaker at the district, the report should be presented and fully explained by the model program manager and on-site coordinator so corrective measures can be taken with pests and conducive conditions.

9. Train the trainers (Appendix A): Steps 8, 9 and 10 usually are conducted at the same time, normally during a three-day visit by the implementation team. This phase – education – is the beginning of actual IPM implementation in the pilot school. We invite (actually insist that) the pest control contractor, technicians, local change agents (Extension, regulatory and local activist – if known) and the designated on-site coordinator to join us during our technical assessment. These people are responsible for implementing change in the system, so this walk-through training is extremely important. However, it is equally important to use this opportunity to develop a good working relationship with all parties involved. We become less teachers and more mentors for these individuals whom we hope will become educators/diagnosticians. This networking is extremely valuable for real-time program troubleshooting. It develops a conduit for moving information we need via e-mail, phone and already-produced materials (fact sheets, newsletters, websites, etc.).

10. Train the school staff adopters: During the last phase of the assessment visit we conduct training for staff (custodial, kitchen, maintenance, etc.), and if possible faculty (including, if we are lucky, the principal), in each school pilot location. The subject matter is pests, pest inducing situations, preventative measures and possible remedial action. Most of all we explain what IPM is, what their current actions mean to pest management and that we are asking them to "do what you are doing now, just think bugs." All the local trainers who just completed their own walk-through training with us are expected to attend. If we communicate effectively, these local trainers actually begin to teach at this point. The best way to learn is to teach, and staff begin to view the program as opportunity for professional improvement. We have learned that this communication works best when we view all staff as professionals and genuinely treat them that way.

11. Monitor (Appendix B): The on-site coordinator monitors schools at least monthly, and if possible, other team members – particularly the pest control contractor – do so as well. They use a variety of methods (traps, staff interviews, visual inspection, etc.) to monitor for the presence of pests and pest-conducive conditions. After discussion with the team pest management professionals, team members facilitate recommendations for preventative measures and possible remedial action at each pilot school. They should be accompanied by senior staff (head custodian, cook, etc.) of each school. If the principal tags along, that's gravy.

12. Introduce: In the initial stages of the pilot program usually only those who are responsible for the school facility are introduced to and educated in the ways of IPM. Soon, though, it becomes important for the remainder of the school community to be introduced to IPM. In this step we initiate a mass media awareness campaign for teachers, administrators, parents and students — the untrained community. If possible, and with the permission of the district, we use local newspapers, but most definitely we use school newsletters and offer to present the program at faculty meetings, school board meetings and to parent-teacher organizations. This stage is critical in garnering support for continuation and expansion, and it also begins the IPM training process for this segment of the community.

13. Newsletters (Appendix E): Unlike the standard school newsletter, this medium is specific to pest management. Ideally, the whole school community is the audience, but normally the district administration finds it cumbersome and expensive to disseminate such information further than the school facility itself. Thus, it is distributed to faculty and staff and posted in appropriate areas of the schools. Some districts include information about their IPM program on their websites. The Monroe County Community School Corporation has developed a website dedicated to its IPM program in hopes that not only will it benefit their school community, but also other school communities throughout the country that wish to use the IPM innovation.

The "Pest Press" first defines IPM and what it means to the school community. It usually addresses a pest of the month, explains why the pest is attracted to the school and tells how to prevent it from infesting the school. It also can include the status of the IPM program, recognize folks who are helping make it work and present short "bug facts" about simple biology insects in general. The key to this newsletter seems to be that whatever information on pest management is provided, it should relate to what is going on in readers' homes. Bingo.

14. Mid-term evaluation (Appendix C): Halfway through the pilot program the implementation team conducts a mid-term evaluation. Basically it is a reassessment of the pilot school program, pest problems and pesticide use that compares IPM results to pre-program conditions, evaluates progress and addresses any new problems. This is a fairly in-depth document that points out progress and problems, with recommendations (action items) to solve those problems. It needs to be disseminated promptly to all those who signed the MOU, then reported back to the school. More often than not, problems at this point are not pest infestations, but rather conducive conditions resulting from human behavior. This is where MOU agreements, which apportioned specific responsibilities to each team member, can be used to help get folks to hold up their end of the program management tasks.

15. Mid-term adjustment meeting: In this step the IPM model program manager should communicate with local implementers to explain the mid-term evaluation recommendations. Ideally this is a face-to-face meeting that explains results of the mid-term evaluation and how the partners can adjust for program improvement. Program adjustments need to be implemented quickly and there should be a scheduled follow-up for each action item. The IPM program manager should elicit the school's response to issues brought up in the evaluation. One common issue we have noticed is the need to improve the work orders process so that facility repair (door sweeps, torn screens, structural cracks, etc.) can be expedited.

16. Handholding. Handholding or nurturing is a natural step during the implementation process. This step is really the IPM program manager's follow-up to implement mid-term recommendations by using a multi-media communication to continue education, and overcome administrative hurdles. You must take them by the hand and walk them through the implementation process because local school implementers often are not sure what happens next. Fact is, IPM implementation to most of them is like a walk in the dark — scary. The more experienced team members need to be on call for more training, more one-on-one inspections and more listening to find out why conducive conditions are not being remediated. Handholding is for all audiences, even the implementation team.

While it's a nurturing process, handholding also is a time for the district to analyze whether or not internalizing Pest Control Operator functions will work. The IPM program manager should introduce this concept to administrators. Based on the district's relationship with its contractor, and the contractor's ability and willingness to partner for real IPM, it might be time to wean the district from the contractor type of management. The district should reevaluate its PCO contract if there is one.

17. Integrate the Pest Management Professional into the model and specific IPM standards: Once the relationship with the exterminator-turned Pest Management- Professional is defined (internal, external, even a combination) the team should spend time working with and emphasizing real IPM with the PCO and the school district. I called this professionalization, whereby the district will:

- Recognize what a quality pest manager is and what a reasonable workload for that person should be.
- Standardize uniform training requirements and joint in-service training for any pest manager.
- Professionalize by upscaling qualifications and compensation to industry standards.
- Centralize by combining and internalizing pest management responsibilities focusing on the school as the unit of operation rather than the program area (food service, grounds, and facilities).

This entire process can be accomplished by ensuring that the school district and its Pest Management Professional are continuously exposed to professional meetings and publications about quality pest management, and that they be made aware of the opportunity for continuing education credits provided by Extension IPM specialists.

18. Final evaluation (Appendix C): This is an evaluation of the program in terms of how the goals of the funding agency were met using a comparison of the baseline, midterm and end of program data. We compare costs, pests, pest-conducive conditions, pesticide use and exposure, and finally the attitudes of the adopting school community. We detail what action items from the mid-term evaluation have been implemented or not, and why. The report goes to all members of the implementation team and then to the school district. When the report does get to the designated decisionmaker in the district, the report should be presented and fully explained by the model program manager and on-site coordinator. The report addresses the percent increase or decrease in costs, pests and pesticide use, program progress and recommendations.

19. District Expansion: Upon a successful evaluation — demonstrated significant decrease in pests, pesticide use, and with no significant increase in cost — the IPM program manager then needs to propose a district-wide IPM program for the participating school district. The IPM program manager must provide an analysis of costs and timeline for implementation. He/she must be able to propose a strategic plan for this implementation, and if need be, propose possible sources of funding. I normally develop this proposal with my implementation team, including the State Lead Agency, the state's IPM Extension Specialist and the USEPA Regional Office prior to presenting to the school district. A standard plan includes funding options, a strategy for expansion (larger districts usually need to implement progressively rather than all at once), personnel requirements (those acting as professional pest managers), training requirements and options and even a public relations campaign. An additional strategy is to assemble a committee of parents who will move expansion forward. Parents have clout. Combined with a committee, their involvement can make a significant contribution.

20. Reward: By recognizing the success of its IPM program, confirmation comes home to the school community and local implementers that they made the right decision in diffusing IPM. Rewards can take the form of award plaques, certificates and positive media exposure. We usually send letters of congratulation to the school district and Extension or entomology department administrators with copies to deans, state agency directors and sometimes the governor's office. These letters congratulate the school district and announce recognition of its efforts in an agreed-upon-in-advance press conference. The key words are, "...for your efforts to protect the children of the state of ...." It works great!

21. Area-Wide Expansion: Your greatest resource for area-wide expansion is the successful program and the local team that worked with you. Use these peers (school facility managers, Pest Management Professional, Extension specialists, etc., from the successful program to get the next group on board. I suggest implementing the Hometown and Coalition models for expansion. They're discussed at the end of this chapter.

22. Report: Prepare Final Compliance Narrative for the funding agency, national press and publication for technical peers.

Lesson 11: Newton's Second Law of Thermodynamics

Without the input of energy, all things tend toward a greater state of entropy (disorder). School districts need to maintain inertia to keep the IPM ball rolling or people will tend to return to pesticides and behaviors conducive to pests.

School districts and their Pest Management Professionals must be careful not to REACT to pest problems (that is, lazy), but to be more proactive. By doing so, they establish a schedule for assessing every school over a reasonable period of time, making sure pest presses are being distributed and that they are spending more time working with staff. Spraying pesticides is not acceptable without documentation, and is not a preventive measure.

It is obvious that this 22-step process requires intensive communication and partnership. It is based on sound pest management as practiced by national experts, but also on the fundamentals of public management that addresses program implementation, politics, and resource acquisition and use. School districts in Alabama, Arizona, California, Florida, Indiana, Ohio and three Native American communities use this model to implement IPM. Policy adoption and faculty/staff education programs are in place in all the districts. Most of the districts that have implemented the model have internalized pest management operations and no longer use regular contracted services. The average pesticide reduction has been 90%, with a similar reduction in pest problems. Each team that adopted the Monroe IPM Model has developed statewide education programs to develop model peer implementers for its state under different supported agreements with the State Lead Agency. Further, each team has participated in programs with, or for, its state's Professional Pest Management Association and/ or Association of School Business Officials. Last, implementation teams reviewed the impacts and shortcomings, made recommendations for model improvement and expansion, and named the model.

A Lame IPM Model?

Nearly all participants in our model evaluation meeting agreed (with me leading the pack) that the "Lame IPM Model", though humorous, sounded too strange, and since it was originally implemented in the Monroe County, Indiana we should keep it simple. Henceforth, our model was to be the Monroe IPM Model. Because of the success of this model and subsequent recognition (built into the Monroe IPM Model), all change agents not only recognized the importance of and required management techniques related to IPM in schools, but also that IPM could actually be implemented in schools without onerous mandates or fiscal upset. Further, these IPM implementers were now willing to consider similar programs for childcare facilities. They (particularly Cooperative Extension and school administrators) strongly felt they benefited from positive exposure in the news and USEPA recognition of their efforts by their superiors. It is always nice for your bosses to recognize there is importance to working on behalf of children.

The IPM implementers felt that complexity (22 steps!) is definitely a negative attribute of this model and of IPM (as a technology cluster) in general. Culprits included the required amounts and types of communication and nurturing. However, simplifying the process could decrease the abundance of positive attributes, particularly the ability of the model to be tested and observed by the adopting school district. Obviously, increased attention to communication should mitigate much of this complexity, as will the increase in numbers of demonstrations around the nation. Many of our implementers felt the model needs to be more considerate of day-to-day operations (including how work-orders are developed) at the schools, and the degree of staff turnover at schools (especially urban schools). For instance, negotiating time away from work for staff in schools has been problematic. In most cases, proper planning, with plenty of lead time, has introduced a greater degree of comfort to this issue. Newsletter production needs to be simplified for school administrators. We now offer them pre-written newsletters on an IPM school website to solve this problem.

Our change agent audience described problems associated with adopters pursuant to this model (obtaining past pest/pesticide use records for baseline data development, engaging state pest management associations and obtaining a more binding commitment for participating school districts), but the audience suggested few improvements for the model. All agreed that school principals are a key resource and should be co-opted at a very early stage in the process. Our audience suggested involving pest control contractors to a greater degree; however, most felt that there had to be a genuine expression of cooperation from the contractors for this to occur. The Monroe IPM Model is a DEMAND-driven model. I am convinced that professional service providers will respond to their customers when those customers are able to say (demand) what they want. Implementers of school IPM recognized that on a national level a number of management tools must be used in order to successfully diffuse IPM in schools nationwide. Those tools include information dissemination (websites, technical manuals), provider (pest control contractor) education and university research and verification/certification programs. However, when the implementers I worked with (during the development of this model to demonstrate IPM in schools) met, they proposed only two basic recommendations for how this model could be diffused nationally. They follow here.

The Hometown Proposal: This proposal allows university entomology departments to access non-competitive funds for a departmental team to implement the Monroe IPM Model in the immediate vicinity of the university. This two-year grant requires the implementing entity to sign an MOU with the USEPA, State Lead Agency and the hometown school district. The second year of funding is contingent on successful implementation of first-year processes. To my knowledge, there is no existing model for this program. Perhaps Auburn University's is similar, but unfortunately most academicians are not coordinated or motivated enough to cooperate on such a community program. That's too bad, seeing that even entomologists have children in public schools. If there are any evangelical department heads out there, please call me, because I know this proposal could work.

Coalition Proposal: This proposal uses Monroe IPM Model adopters to implement statewide diffusion of IPM in schools, in combination with change agents and funding agencies. Essentially it is a project that uses the initial school district (after one complete year of district-wide implementation) and the implementation team to initiate the Monroe IPM Model for a coalition of school districts, as a springboard to statewide expansion. This requires that the regional or state IPM implementation manager form and chair a taskforce for the expansion of IPM in schools. The coalition should include school pilot program participants, administrators, professional pest manager(s), public health officials and children's health advocates in coalition with selected suburban rural and intercity school districts (one to two pilot schools/district). The administrative training is to be coordinated by the initial pilot program school district and faculty/staff trainings conducted jointly by peers and Extension specialists. Other aspects of this proposal follow the 22 model steps. However, several managerial aspects have been added so state program coordinators can sustain their program.

Dawn Gouge at the University of Arizona partnered with me to implement a coalition model in Arizona in 2003. I got my old employer — the Arizona Department of Environmental Quality — to talk Region 9, USEPA, Office of Pesticide programs, into funding this as a children's environmental health initiative. Dawn talked Stan Peterson with Kyrene into chairing our coalition partners. The coalition was forged among strategically picked school communities and various change agents including the Arizona Department of Environmental Quality, Arizona Department of Health, Arizona Structural Pest Control Commission, the University of Arizona, Department of Entomology, the USEPA and private sector Pest Management Professionals.

Our IPM support team, made up of many of the folks I have introduced you to in this book, is implementing IPM as we do with the standard Monroe IPM Model. The team is training local IPM on-site coordinators, facility managers, faculty and staff; demonstrating workable IPM techniques and people management innovations for the incorporation of those techniques (e.g., pest sighting logbooks, clutter control, etc.); developing and disseminating pest presses; conducting audits of pest management costs and pesticide use; conducting periodic evaluations of program progress; and doing face-to-face debriefings of decisionmakers about the mitigation of risk to the school community. This is a coalition intended to facilitate the statewide adoption of school Integrated Pest Management in the absence of an appropriately funded mandate.

It is time for us to move beyond school-district-by-school-district implementation to a more regional approach that uses school administrators to create the "critical mass" that will allow verifiable IPM to become the norm in school environmental management. We do recognize that most school districts in the U.S. do not have the volume (at least 15 schools per district) and must contract with a Pest Management Professional. Therefore, we must develop an ethical, workable and profitable contract model so these educators/diagnosticians can become full partners in implementing IPM in their school districts.

The differences between the Coalition Model and our standard district Monroe IPM Model are that the Coalition version:

- Develops 10, strategically picked core school districts that are required to meet quarterly to provide quality control, assurance and support.
- Maintains a single, monthly pest press publication that can be modified and owned by each participating school district.
- Maintains only one pilot school per core district school.
- Transfers leadership to school managers and relegates state IPM program managers to advisor and coordinator roles.
- Establishes a business plan and training program to utilize specific private sector, pest management professionals.
- Works with Cooperative Extension and State Lead Agencies (under FIFRA) to develop statewide workshops (upgrading training and certification) for adopting school personnel and contractors.

Our coalition project currently is in the process of implementing the Monroe IPM Model in 11 Arizona school districts that have not adopted verifiable IPM programs. These school districts represent rural, border, inner-city, suburban and Indian Lands school districts. The over-arching goal of this coalition is to establish a successful and transferable national model for protecting our school community from pests and pesticides.

The Arizona IPM Coalition will "insert" technologies proven to protect the indoor air quality of Arizona's school students. With any luck we will be able to teach the USEPA so it can use existing structures to diffuse environmental innovations like IPM as a network and a mechanism to provide a truly safer learning environment for our school communities. That beats reinventing the wheel every time they come up with a new way to improve their environmental quality...Stay tuned.

Chapter Twelve – Resources for Success - "Comrades and Conspirators"

In this chapter I will open with an act of academic heresy. We in academe are taught to document, verify and publish. Nice stuff, and it is part of my religion. However, I know too few in academe – universities – who really contribute much beyond their protected system. It is far too comfortable to study an effect rather than effecting change. By all means, study — gather data, analyze data, and verify — but DO SOMETHING WITH IT! Of course, effecting change is risky business — change is near and dear. Publishing in obscure journals or trade magazines and presenting to scientific societies and industry groups might earn you tenure (the gold ring of the academic), but you need to "get your hands dirty", as my mentor, Leon Moore, used to tell me when I was in cotton IPM. Give, rather than take, or at least be a risk taker.

The bottom line is that nothing breeds success like success. Whereas the USDA IPM program seems to fund only the gathering of information about whether we should be implementing IPM in schools (gee, I wonder who is controlling them?), those of us in the trenches are "just doing it". Again, thanks, Al Greene, for your 1996 admonishment to our group of school IPM implementers about what "the right thing" is when it comes to children and pest management.

When I teach program implementation to public management students, I tell them that three questions must be asked and answered for the successful implementation of any program: 1) What action is to be taken? 2) Who will take that action? and 3) Does that entity have the resources to take action? Based on previous chapters, you have a very good idea of what action needs to be taken. Now I want to be more specific regarding Who will take that action (many of these folks will be familiar) and what resources they need to take that action.

The IPM Implementation Team

In the broadest sense, the best resource you have at hand is your product —successful pilot schools/districts and their new believers! They best represent the action that should be taken. That's why we call it a model. But pest management is also people management, and I rely on people to be the successful implementers of the Monroe IPM Model. I rely on people every time I am asked to expand IPM into school districts that don't practice it.

These people come in a variety of flavors. All are quite valuable and often interchangeable in their individual abilities to address the diffusion process outlined in the previous chapter. In this chapter I describe several different professional types a good manager might want on his/her team for the successful implementation of IPM in schools. As a very hands-on manager, I believe the fewer the better when it comes to efficient teamwork. Fortunately, many of these professional types can multi- task, thereby typically reducing the actual implementation team to seven or eight individuals.

Regional or National Team Members

- **Program coordinator (administrator, director, grand pooh-bah)**

This individual (or in some cases one or two co-directors) develops funding (normally based on competitive bids), initiates each step of the implementation process, facilitates TEAM communication, sets agendas, organizes training, conducts the first and last evaluation, provides management recommendations, plays politics and writes the reports. Yep, that's me. And I can assure you about one-third of the way into each project, I wish I was just crawling around in custodial closets looking for mouse droppings. In truth, I believe, from experience, that almost any of the team members I describe below can assume this management — if they are true believers and their bosses allow them.

This is a true managerial position responsible for the three basic management functions that any administrator must competently address:

program, political and resource management. This person does not have to be an entomologist, but had better know IPM and how it applies to a specific topic area (i.e., schools vs. cotton fields). It also helps to have a few Gary Larson cartoons on your wall.

Strategic communication planning is Job One for the program coordinator:

1) Know the management situation (e.g., convincing participants to sign the MOU);
2) know your audience (agency reps vs. university entomologists vs. school district facility managers vs. community activists vs. school principals vs. custodians ..... you get my drift);
3) know your most effective messages (tone, wording, timing etc.);
4) know the most effective ways (including news media) to send that message (e-mail, newsletter, TV, face-to-face, etc.); and
5) know how best to obtain and evaluate feedback to determine what you have to do next.

Like any effective team leader (administrator), this individual must always do whatever is necessary to allow team members to perform their jobs so they can achieve successful implementation. For this person, people are primary resources. As a team member, partner and friend, I always try to make each individual understand two fundamental messages: "You are the best person for this job", and "Let me know what I can do for you".

However, these specific human resources will always need specific material resources and specific messages to accomplish their specific tasks. I will include what I consider the best message (or mantra) and an example of communications (with some names withheld) I, as the Program Coordinator, use specific to nurturing/motivating/and sometime castigating each human (team) resource.

- **Funding agency representatives**

These entities (e.g., USEPA HQ and/or Regional Office of Pesticide Programs) identify agency expectations, facilitate funding and promote expansion of the program internally. They are bureaucrats. Some are better at taking risks than others. I don't bother to work with the USDA Integrated Pest Management folks anymore, as they won't take any risks to promote school IPM. It is not really their mission. Most of my communication is with the USEPA, Office of Pesticide Programs. Take a look at its mission statement:

"To protect public health and the environment from risks posed by pesticides and promote safer means of pest control."
"One of OPP's main concerns is increased protection for the public, especially for infants and children. OPP seeks to educate consumers, as well as to keep them informed about the risks of pesticides. The health of infants and children has a high priority, since they are more vulnerable to pesticides than adults. OPP has taken extra measures in order to protect children from risk."

The two best messages to send this group are: "Your agency has a mandate to implement IPM in schools, thereby protecting children's environment health" and "Please allow us to help you fulfill that mandate and give you credit for doing so".

To a Regional EPA Office of Pesticide Programs manager (from me) –

"I want to express my gratitude for your recognition of those that have been attempting to create a safer learning environment for our nation's children. Per your recognition there are many professionals who believe school IPM to be worthy of efforts above and beyond their normally evaluated job responsibilities - primarily because, as Dr. Al Green phrased it, "it is the right thing to do". I am grateful, not only for this recognition, but for the extraordinary efforts of particular individuals in the USEPA that have made the implementation of school IPM possible. I know that a significant portion of this effort is sometimes "under the table" and at the risk of "rocking the boat" - Thank You.

Finally, as a rogue entomologist that also teaches management communication at IU, I want to recognize the quality management of "rewarding implementers". However, I must also express my sincere disappointment in what must be the lack of correct decision making, or caring in the Public Affairs area of your agency. Where, there seems to be no commitment towards a coordinated effort to publicize school IPM whenever possible. The fact that most of the recipients of this award deserved this coordinated effort by your PIOs is minor (and very forgivable) compared to the larger missed opportunity. The big story is what EPA is doing for children (and without specific legislated mandate) through this recognition - AND your "media flaks" missed it. Gee, I guess I just blew my chances at anymore grant money...but I ain't giving back the plaque."

Excerpts of a letter for an USEPA Administrator (from me) –

"The Office of Pesticide Programs has been at the forefront of developing national tools for the implementation of IPM in schools and is promoting the voluntary, national expansion of IPM in schools with committed partners. We feel a real opportunity exists to establish a successful and transferable pollution prevention/risk reduction program that can move beyond the "school district by school district" implementation to a more regional approach by supporting the expansion of this current project... This program can be a real winner for all involved in terms of program achievement and public recognition. Please let me know when we can discuss this issue – I will look forward to your participation."

Without question, the program coordinator must rely on agencies like this to obtain funding. And believe me; they must abide by the rules of competitive bidding for grant proposals. As a former government official I strongly believe that one can have an ethical relationship among grant administrators and recipients or prospective recipients of public monies. In fact, a degree of professional intimacy allows for better communication, and therefore, a clearer understanding of goals and objectives. I do not go begging for grants. I know that the most productive way government can dispense funding is to partner with professionals, who not only write proposals, but who have a successful track record, have transparent operations and are inclusive in the process of implementation...people who don't just know snippets of information but can prove they get results in an ethical manner and will share credit with their partners.

Excerpt from the Navajo project Request for Proposals to the USEPA -

"What we are proposing is that the ("Monroe") model be extended to tribal school communities on the Navajo Reservation (New Mexico and Arizona).

The successful extension of the ("Monroe") model will initiate a proven pesticide reduction program to two fundamental audiences- the school community and to change agents (State Lead Agencies, Cooperative Extension, PCOs, and future pest management professionals). It will provide education through training, demonstrate technological and program planning innovations, develop and disseminate outreach materials, conduct audits of pesticide use, cost and exposure outlining tangible progress for the mitigation of risk to the tribal school community, and is designed to be transferable to other tribal school communities.

Finally, the network to begin these pilot programs has been developed. We have obtained provisional approval from the key change agents in Arizona and on the Navajo Reservation (including USEPA, OPP state program managers). While this pilot will access nationally recognized resources (personnel and educational materials), these resources will be adapted for maximum effectiveness in this particular cultural situation."

The Program Coordinator must develop a strong and comfortable relationship with funding agency representatives. They have their requirements and you must help them meet those requirements. I communicate with these folks at least weekly to update and nurture. Many of my colleagues actually wait for their representatives to contact them. Big mistake! If you want a person to act like a bureaucrat, treat them like one. I don't. I treat them (maybe long ago they joined the agency because they wanted to make a difference) like partners who do make a difference, and they will, in terms of providing funding and their bully pulpit.

A short e-mail to my contact in the agency –

"Yesterday it came to me that our last several calls have been somewhat depressing. I want to remind you (and myself) that we have made a difference - to children, real pest management professionals, child advocates, and ourselves. We prove that real partners can change the world on a shoe string. No matter what narrow sighted, turf bound, officials might or might not do - what we have done will continue to make a difference. Let them play their games - and follow us, and wish they could make a difference too. Too bad they don't realize it just takes force of will. Have a nice day."

- **Pest management professional –**

These are people who get to have all the fun, from an entomological point of view. They conduct technical assessments, provide technical recommendations and help conduct training for staff and local Pest Control Operators. Sometimes this individual doubles as one of the IPM Coordinators (peer or on-site), or comes from the Cooperative Extension ranks. Either way, they are diagnosticians and educators. My folks simply are the best people I can convince to help, and afford, as contractors. They're guys like Bobby Corrigan, Mike Lindsey and Larry Pinto. They are the on the top of the mountain when it comes to qualifying as diagnosticians and educators.

This is a special partnership. As with the partnership of marriage, we rely on each other, learn from each other and occasionally bang heads — normally because of my uncompromising attitude toward those who don't practice real IPM. These guys are in the business of customer service and are careful not to alienate their food processing, structural and grocery store chain customers who pay a hell of a lot more than I do. Further, they are somewhat fraternal with regard to their industry. That said, these guys know the real thing and practice it. They mostly just roll their eyes when I go off on "the way it should be".

I listen to how they say technical assessments should be done, what should be reported and identify specific trouble spots. Not surprisingly, trouble spots are more people management-related than physical. A seasoned pest management professional recognizes human tendencies that result in pest-conducive conditions and usually has great suggestions for dealing with those humans.

When our model programs are completed, the pest management professional has ensured:

- a detailed technical assessment of each school;
- priority and long-term recommendations to address conducive conditions;
- references for the remediation of these conditions;
- recommendations specific to any pest infestation
- one-on-one training for the school staff that accompany them during their assessment
- suggestions for group training, program management; and
- on-call availability for any conditions or infestations that occur at the pilots schools for the duration of the program.

They provide our team with excellent entertainment, pest management education, political support, and suggestions for working with those in their industry.

Excerpt from an e-mail sent by a Professional Pest Manager expressing his concern about the lack of follow-through from the school district administration and the school staff –

"Great email report! First, I will put it on my calendar to call you around 8:30 on Monday morning - if that is ok? Second, as we develop more data regarding pest management at the pilots schools (i.e. - paint a picture) we can take it to (their) administration and ask if they are serious or not. That's why it is nice to have (a strong activist group) partnering on this one.... FYI, I did let USEPA know that if they do not have plans/resources for making the project work, it will fail."

- **Peer facilities manager –**

This person conducts the management and cost audit, facilitates administrative communication and tells the "IPM story" from an insider point of view. I have mentioned John Carter at our Bloomington school district and Stan Peterson in Tempe. In many ways they say what most of the rest of the team says to the school district staff. Except... those folks actually listen to John and Stan because they are of their own beleaguered fraternity. Day in, day out, they do more with less. In this respect these guys are the preferred medium to transmit our messages.

When it comes to what management expects to be taking place in the schools and the costs of pest management, this team member is critical. He/she knows what questions to ask and where to get the answers. Without the baseline data these folk generate, we cannot prove to the school district decisionmakers and funding agency representatives that real IPM does what we say it will.

I often use these team members as examples of the tangible rewards to adopting IPM — and they fully deserve them. They become the topics of newspaper articles, award recipients and guest speakers at conferences. Always surprising to me is that these very busy individuals become our true disciples of school IPM. It seems they, like other public officials, genuinely enjoy the positive lights of IPM. And those are much needed lights in the school district's complaint department.

- **Peer IPM coordinator –**

Some school districts have their own pest management unit — most of the time they call it Pest Control. Too often they are convinced that they are really practicing IPM. Most often they are not. This is where guys like Jerry Jochim come in. As the IPM Coordinator in Bloomington and a former district maintenance staffer, Jerry is more credible to Pest Control Operators than I or anyone else on the team. He assists in technical assessment and training, facilitates staff communication and can tell the IPM story from an insider point of view.

The program coordinator's job is to make sure this individual has the necessary resources (in terms of training, presentation and information dissemination) to conduct these special tasks:

> **Diagnostician training** – You have already been introduced to Jerry. His training was from scratch. Bobby and I took Jerry with us on every school visit, reviewed certification materials for his license with him and made sure he understood the difference between becoming certified and practicing real IPM. We made sure he got to practice the technical aspects of his trade — identification, monitoring, conducive condition remediation and, when needed, infestation elimination. We supplied him with the tools for that application: references for pest identification (Internet and hard copy), monitoring traps, inspection tools (special flashlights, pry bars, hand lens, mirrors, etc.) and pest control tools, both mechanical and chemical.

> **Educator training and information** – Jerry had to learn *what* to teach and *how* to teach it to his specific audiences. He transformed from a member of the congregation into the preacher. This is real hearts and minds stuff, but he is one of them and it works! Further, we made sure he had newsletters, websites and mass media articles to leave with those he educated (see Appendix E).

Local Team Members

- **State Lead Agency (SLA – state Agricultural Departments, Structural Pest Control Commissions, and Departments of Environmental Quality) –**

This state regulatory agency provides local funding, regulatory hammer, and facilitates industry communication and training. Most importantly, it should assume responsibility for statewide expansion with Cooperative Extension. Of course, the problem is the agency often is co-opted by or controlled by industry. The real work for the program coordinator is to empower this group, and it deserves it.

Most of this is political management. These are political animals who look good if the governor feels good about what they are doing. I will explain the policy of school IPM more fully in the next chapter, but know there is a political tug-of-war between children's environmental health activists and the pest control industry that influences decisionmakers on this issue. If the SLA is allowed to feel that IPM in schools is a win-win situation for children's environmental health, and at least for the niche group of real pest management professionals in the state, the SLA will be a responsible resource. Further, the SLA is authorized by the USEPA, Office of Pesticide Programs, to implement FIFRA. Therefore, the program coordinator must minimize the political risks, provide maximum reward and ask little up-front participation from this team member.

In our MOU we require the SLA and/or Cooperative Extension representative to provide:

- Onsite coordination and communication about information dissemination in your program area.
- Data gathering/sharing with regard to existing or ongoing economic and pest surveys that address pest management in schools.
- Willingness to coordinate activities with other states (depending on travel funding).
- Tailor-made version of this program to their state, however within the confines of the Monroe IPM Model parameters.
- Bi-monthly communication with a PESP Partnership representative.
- Attendance and participation in at least one training session and one on-site inspection.

Cooperative Extension –

The Cooperative Extension IPM Specialist or Agent provides local situation analysis as it pertains to common pests, pest management and professional pest managers. The agent also must assist with all forms of assessment and training, and should be responsible for statewide expansion with the SLA.

These people are academicians and the most important thing the program coordinator can do for them is to make sure their bosses at the university are happy. At best, their bosses want to "do the right thing", but will settle for program recognition, funding and peer-reviewed publications for their employees so they can get them tenure. At worst, their bosses want these scientists to "extend" their scientific expertise to a paying industry and not rock the boat.

Either way, the IPM specialist or urban entomologist knows the most up-to-date technical aspects of pest management. I usually learn a great deal from them in this regard. In my opinion they are the perfect folks to lead the state's child-sensitive community into a fully implemented IPM program. Unfortunately, I will remind you that these fine scientists are often woefully deficient when it comes to management skills, tend to be profoundly risk-averse and sometimes act as though they can casually own IPM without being leaders in its implementation. I must admit I do take some pleasure in reminding them I used to be in their club, then educating them in the fact that there is a whole non-USDA world out there. They usually are welcoming, but unsure where I am coming from and uncomfortable with my ex-patriot demeanor. I love their profession and respect them.

- **The Activist –**

This person stimulates action from the local school administration and provides checks/balances and local support. Without doubt, these team members are the most controversial of any of our implementers because, by nature, they are loose cannons. They often have a no-pesticide agenda, are accustomed to being mistreated by government types, have a hard time trusting and are impatient. I admire and respect them and have learned the hard way that verifiable implementation of real IPM is not going to work without them.

The only way the program coordinator can keep the activist from attacking the program is to include this person as a full partner. Most other members of the team are scared to death of activists. As mentioned in previous chapters, public officials are accustomed to working with industry people who use familiar language. The fact is, industry people are simply just activists with whom public officials are comfortable. Thus, the program coordinator must facilitate a degree of trust and comfort with this team member and other teams at the same time. Communication and developing what Rosemary O'Leary calls a "co-production environmental ethic" (O'Leary, et al., 1999) accomplish this goal.

Simply put, a co-production environmental ethic comes about when members of the community or team co-produce a solution to an environmental problem — a win-win solution. Real IPM as I have described it, communicated correctly, does address pests and pesticides in child-sensitive facilities in a win-win fashion.

By and large, I ask activist team members to assist when necessary and to accept credit with the rest of the team. They need to be privy to most communications with the school district, and invited to planning meetings, program evaluation meetings and press conferences. When school administrators or other public officials who are local team members become unresponsive, activists can communicate with them, and believe me, they swing a big stick when they want to. Normally, just their presence keeps administrators in line. Their ability to reward local team members, using their bully pulpit, can produce tangible positive benefits for all involved.

- **On-site IPM coordinator –**

This is where the rubber meets the road in terms of diagnosing and education. The on-site IPM coordinator:

- Conducts bi-weekly or monthly, technical and even political management assessments of status of conducive conditions;
- maintains the monitoring plan developed in the initial technical assessments;
- recommends and monitors actions for pest infestations and educates the school, administration, faculty and staff (particularly about conducive conditions and pest logs);
- is responsible for distribution of newsletters and pesticide application notification; and
- most important of all, maintains frequent communication with the program coordinator. On-site coordinators are the eyes, ears and voice of the implementation team.

Make no mistake, these are real, crawl-on-their-bellies, bug tasting professional pest managers. Sometimes they double as the national pest management team member, or are locals who always enjoy working with our national experts. But, what they have to bring to the party is:

1) Know-how — whether they had it coming into the program or can comfortably access it while on the job. Dawn Gouge, Fudd Graham, Lyn Hawkins, Jerry Jochim, Mike Lindsey, I and later Larry Schmiets, Carl Olson and Carl Martin have all acted in this capacity.

2) An incredible ability to infect others with the IPM spirit. I believe we all can tell you that this is the most demanding but enjoyable part of implementing the IPM model in schools.

> **An evaluation report for the Clark County Schools On-site IPM Coordinator -** Lyn Hawkins has developed and utilized considerable expertise implementing IPM in the pilot schools and has been the key component in our training program – especially regarding the educational component to the staff and administrators. Not enough can be said about Mr. Hawkins' incredible communication and teaching techniques. A real pro.
>
> He reviewed the technical recommendations provided by Dr. Corrigan and assisted the pilot schools in their understanding of the remediation of these conducive conditions. He documented the status of the remediation of conducive conditions by the pilot schools, and developed and implemented an aggressive ant management program for Diskin Elementary School with the assistance of Drs. Corrigan, Lame and Smith. Further, Lyn concentrated pest management activities at Ranch High School in the cafeteria complex (kitchen, dock, cafeteria, storage rooms, and teachers lounge) so as to demonstrate conducive condition remediation and rodent control. Finally, he scheduled the development, release and distribution of three more monthly newsletters (issue topics - ants, roaches, and mice/spiders respectively) with Marc Lame, Eddie Giron, and the pilot school principals in the Clark County School District.

On-site IPM coordinators work best when they can easily schedule visits to their pilot schools and spend whatever time necessary to diagnose and educate. Unfortunately, these individuals cannot always reside in the school district, so their travel schedules need to be fairly flexible. On at least three projects I coordinated, our on-site IPM coordinator lived in an adjacent state. It was not ideal, but quite workable. Why? Because this person had adequate travel funding, knew his job and had other team members as resources.

Excerpts from typical e-mail communication with one of our on-site IPM coordinators – The Great Pumpkin – Mike Lindsey in Tempe Arizona –

> **To Marc:** Monitoring Traps at Cielo -
>
> | Office area (4 traps) | Kitchen area (4 traps) |
> |---|---|
> | 1 roach (1 adult) | 2 roaches (1 adult, 1 nymph) |
> | 4 crickets | 9 mothflies |
> | 1 firebrat | 1 scorpion (Centuroides) |
>
> A Black Widow hatch in the cooling towers area will be cleaned up with a shop vac. Silicon sealant will be used in maintenance storage to reduce cricket harborage - pipes coming through walls, slab and wall separation, etc., etc..
>
> Marc (you rascally person) please call Stan on a land line - his e-mail is KAPOOT! - to confirm the Nov. 1 meeting. Everything is Jake, but you two need to hable!
>
> Dawn (you equally rascally person) we have a request from Ms. Jody Pfeffer for a classroom visitation Oct. 12 - Grades 1 & 2 -Paloma. We need to hable. I am and will continue to be, The Great Pumpkin
>
> **To The Great Pumpkin:** Yummie report. I am assuming these counts were pre-treatment (roaches)? Mothflies- something stinks (in the sink/drain - unused since?). What is the status on (the contactor) and sewer/slabs? Let's get the ground cover squared away while the weather is warm (113 today?). Marc

Yep, Mike obviously enjoys his work. Gotta love a guy who thinks scorpions are pets.

These folks are highly motivated IPM implementers. However, their frame of reference is as educators and diagnosticians not program managers. They hate writing reports even more than I do. It is critical that the Program Coordinator communicate with the implementation team — particularly during mid-term and final assessments. Assessments and the school district decisionmaker debriefing must follow outline program progress and determine the outcome of implementation. The following e-mail exchange is an example of how I communicate with my team and the guidelines that I needed to clarify so those team members could achieve the success we all desired:

Excerpts from my e-mail communication with Program Manager ("co-director") Dawn Gouge and on-site IPM coordinators - January, 2005

And a happy Monday morning to all,

First, I was wondering who was picking up the tab for all the margaritas that folks had during Jerry's visit? Am not sure any work got done, as I got complaints from several bar managers in Central and Southern Arizona regarding drunken IPM folks shining scorpion flashlights in patrons' eyes and crawling under tables looking for pests (likely story).

Seriously, I understand much was accomplished last week and wanted to thank everyone for their hard work. As usual, what we found out was more of what we have to do - faculty/staff trainings, kicking admin. butts, etc. However, it seems that all except Kyrene are moving in the right direction. Further, I believe Tempe Elementary SD is wanting to join the Coalition and it is possible that the PHX Area Catholic School District will join as well - stay tuned.

So, up-coming is the Scottsdale annual audit, Harris at Gilbert?, Paradise Valley initial audit? and the visit by Gregg Smith from Salt Lake City to do Indoor Air Quality (IAQ) interviews - not to mention monthly On-site IPM Coordinator pilot school visits.

Some administrative requests from Marc - one time, fun loving, boy entomologist, latter-day pain in the butt:

1- On-site IPM Coordinators (Olson, Schmeits, Lindsey) and Children's Health Specialist (Martin), and Jerry (I won't tell you what I call him) - Please turn in your January invoices with any reports you have been assigned by Tuesday of next week (the Aztec audit can be included knowing the report will follow). My quarterly reports to Mike Wallace (EPA money launderer) are awaiting your reports. Because our grant period ends in October, I am having much fun securing funding beyond October to support more AZ stuff as well as regional (SW, Rocky Mtn., and NW) projects any of you might be interested in. You can imagine I go to sleep every night just dying to put on my white belt, used car salesman outfit, call bureaucrats and write stimulating government grants such that we can do their job for them. And I teach students here at the U to become one of them?

2- Please review these guidelines regarding what I believe the On-site IPM Coordinator should consider. Clearly we all agree our on-site inspection/reporting/educator standards must be higher than most public school employees and pest control industry folks. Our credibility with Coalition members depends on our field work and on-site implementation to have very little wiggle room at this point in the process. Let me know what you think on this stuff.

I know that Dawn, Jennifer and Jerry are working-up job descriptions and expanded/better guidelines such that we can do a better job developing folks like you in different parts of the country.
• Any visit/audit should be scheduled to include your partner if you are doing team work.
• It is always a good idea to review previous inspection reports before going to do an on-site inspection. If you don't have them ask for them.
• Monthly reports (one page is fine) should address specific progress related to initial/mid-term audits and/or other monthly reports - they should be comparative in terms of progress and informative in terms of status. These reports are not just for me, but are a communication to each pilot school and district decisionmaker regarding progress and suggested tactics.
• Initial, Mid-term and final/annual audits should be very much more like the Harris report (please ask Dawn or me for any previous reports you need). Clearly, we need a detailed, prioritized report when you/we go to the district decisionmakers to get them on board.
• On-site IPM Coordinators should always be accompanied by the pest control tech (am still not willing to say PMP for all the folks out there - it is your job to help them become one), and the head custodian. If you cannot

get this commitment, please notify me or Dawn and we will communicate with whomever.

Please keep in mind the difference between a school district IPM program coordinator and an On-site IPM Coordinator - particularly in terms of reports and communication. Marc

To this point of better team management, Dawn and I in the previous two months had done some great negotiating and planning with regard to coordination and management of the coalition. We were really comfortable about where the coalition (see last page of Chapter 11) was heading. Fact is, we had played a lot of this by ear over the past year, not knowing exactly where it was headed or how to manage it. Sometimes life is like that. In these types of situations (personal or professional) the best thing is to respect, communicate and coordinate and communicate — did I mention communicate?

Dawn convinced me to provide more resources in preparation for our "coalition independence" meeting at which we intended to hand over leadership to coalition members. It was very important that we be allowed to delegate more without burning out the delegates. I felt very strongly we needed to adhere to the following management tasks for Quality assurance/Quality control:

1) Develop AND SHARE a calendar of scheduled initial, mid-term, and reassessments, assessment report due dates AND assessment follow-up meets for the next quarter. I had increased the role of our on-site IPM coordinators to covering 11 core schools districts.
2) Commit to biweekly 1-2 hour communications with our implementation team.
3) Develop monthly coalition member e-mail updates to discuss coalition status.

At that point in Dawn's academic career, her administration was requiring her to demonstrate excellence in what amounted to two full-time positions (extension and research). Therefore, it was extremely important for me to put her time (in the office and the field) foremost in my decisionmaking when determining how to complete the tasks mentioned above. I promised it would require less time and allow more time for her tenure preparation IF we enforced a disciplined schedule of assignments and communication.

- **Current pest manager or contractor** –

These individuals are licensed pest control operators — they can legally apply pesticides. In our model they have the same diagnostician responsibilities as on-site IPM coordinators, but usually do not spend as much "educator" time at report writing and political debriefing. In all the programs I have been involved with, pest control contractors either did not take the time, and/or had no authority to implement proper IPM or educate the school faculty and staff with about pest management. Once given the responsibility, authority (and, if necessary, the training) to become diagnosticians and educators, they essentially become IPM coordinators like Jerry Jochim. Of course the great advantage to retaining such individuals is that you can monitor and train them in the use of pesticides if necessary. They know the physical layout of the school fairly well, and if they are an actual school district employee they usually have much better communication with school staff because they understand the political realities of their work situation.

The key to developing these existing pest managers is to treat them like professionals, making it very clear that real professional pest managers are always in the learning mode. I always learn from these folks, usually in terms of what and where the problems are — not how to effectively address those problems. They often feel threatened by our team in the beginning, but they also normally rise to the occasion if allowed. This allowance can become a political management problem with the next type of team member.

- **District decisionmaker** –

These leaders of the school administration provide political support within the school district and make the decision to expand and provide an organizational structure for expansion. The real and verifiable implementation of IPM in their school district begins and ends with them. Usually, the decisionmakers we work with are either the **Facilities administrator** (who coordinates pest management services, staff training and conducive condition remediation among to custodial and maintenance staff) or the **Food service administrator** who is similar to the facilities administrator, but in the area of food service. Sometimes if we are lucky, the decisionmaker is a member of the school board or the district superintendent.

It is absolutely necessary to understand that it takes years for these administrators to understand what REALLY goes on in their system. I have yet to talk to any school administrator who really knew what was going on with pest management. They will always assure you they are already doing "the right thing". I have been told that all schools in a given district were serviced only by their own "IPM technicians" only to find out that principals in some schools were contracting with local exterminators because they felt the "IPM technicians" were not effective at controlling their mice. Worse, I was told by one school district administrator that they no longer used or contracted exterminators to use pesticides in their schools. Then I found that the district issued cases of over-the-counter pesticides including rat poison, aerosol cans and insecticide foggers. This is why I always try to bring in their peers who understand what they did NOT know when they began the program. Fortunately, these decisionmakers understand what "the right thing" looks like to their school community. It is up to the team to prove to them what the right thing really is.

Of course they want to know that it won't take too much of their time, cost them money, or put them at risk. That's fair. Their plate is full, their budget is pitiful and people regularly take bites out of them. Go to a school board meeting and watch. So we mitigate the risk by providing a model that they can try out in the form of a pilot program We paint a picture of what is really going on in their sphere of responsibility as it pertains to pest management — a plan for district wide implementation in a cost-neutral situation — and offer political support in the form of awards and recognition.

A Press Release for the Auburn City Schools Program - Auburn City Schools and Auburn University to Receive Awards Recognized for Reducing Children's Exposure to Pesticides by 90 Percent

The National Foundation for Integrated Pest Management Education (NFIPME) and the USEPA, Office of Pesticide Programs are honoring Auburn City Schools and the Auburn University's Department of Entomology & Plant Pathology for their efforts in reducing pest infestations and pesticide use by 90 percent in local schools.

A press conference and brief award presentation will be held Friday, April 25, at 10 a.m. at the Auburn City Schools Board Office located at 855 East Samford Avenue in Auburn, Alabama.

The award will be presented to Dr. J. Terry Jenkins, Superintendent of the Auburn City Schools and Dr.

187

Michael Williams, Chair of the Auburn University Department of Entomology & Plant Pathology by Dr. Marc Lame, on behalf of NFIPME.

Auburn City Schools began this program in partnership with the U.S. EPA, the Alabama Department of Agriculture and Industry, and the Auburn University in 2000.

The Austin, Texas-based NFIPME is a non-profit organization dedicated to more effective and environmentally sound pest management practices. Integrated Pest Management (IPM) enhances existing school operations with professional pest management techniques.

The USEPA, Office of Pesticide Programs funds pilot programs throughout the United States to demonstrate the effectiveness of Integrated Pest Management (IPM) in the school environment. Dr. Marc Lame who manages the implementation of many of these programs says, "The best message we can send schools is that IPM is not more on their plate, and they can implement IPM by doing what they are doing now regarding building security, energy management, and sanitation – just think pests. This program is all about education" Further, he states that "Schools end up using IPM because it is the right thing to do for their students."

This children's health protection effort is supported by most federal and state agencies through their effort to provide a safer learning environment for our children. IPM is recognized as one of the most progressive efforts for reducing the risk of pest related illnesses and pesticide exposure to children by national children's health advocacy organizations such as Improving Kids Environment, based in Indianapolis, IN.

- **Principals –**

Most of the public schools we work with have a management system called site-based administration. In other words, the everyday workings within a particular school site are under control of the school principal.

Principals tell the local staff and faculty the way it will be. They control the people and the space to which the school community entrusts its children. In terms of IPM, principals allow either good or bad cultural control in the form of standards for sanitation and clutter. More importantly, they control the flow of information that affects pest-conducive conditions related to sanitation and clutter.

As an audience these, folks are educators who have become the Supreme Being in their professional universe. Objectively, I see their egos and prideful attitudes as huge assets for implementing something good for their charges (students, faculty and staff). The challenge is meeting with them long enough to communicate the positive attributes of IPM. I must admit that these folks scare the hell out of me.

A sample introductory letter to a pilot school principal –

Dear Principal's name,

My name is Marc Lame, and I teach at Indiana University's School of Public and Environmental Affairs (SPEA). I also work under a cooperative agreement with the USEPA Office of Pesticide Programs to implement the risk reduction program known as Integrated Pest Management (IPM) in which your school district has agreed to participate on a trial basis.

During my recent visit I was very impressed by the willingness of your school district to do whatever possible to provide a safe learning environment for your school community, and the high level of environmental management that currently exists. The model program I implement on behalf of the USEPA, "The Monroe IPM Model", is successful in the school environment because cultural and mechanical strategies can be incorporated into the existing custodial and maintenance activities such as sanitation, energy conservation, building security and infrastructure maintenance. This approach has been implemented for more than nine years, and has demonstrated a 90% reduction in pesticide use, and pests/complaints--without significantly increasing staff workload or district expense (normally decreased) in six states and three Arizona Indian Reservations. Please feel free to view our IPM school website, http://www.ipm.mccsc.edu , or discuss this program with any of the school facilities administrators listed on this site.

During this current school year we will provide the required resources needed to increase the implementation of IPM at ?school name? in Elementary School District. These resources will be in the forms of: 1) Personnel (nationally recognized trainers and assessors with experience successfully implementing IPM in schools in other states); 2) educational and implementation information and materials; 3) training school district personnel in your pilot school(s); 4) monitoring station and technical materials; and 5) an "On-site IPM Coordinator" for scheduled monitoring and program implementation.

Implementation team members include your current pest manager, ?PMP name? (as the "On-site IPM Coordinator), Dr. Dawn Gouge (University of Arizona), and me. We will also be coordinating the implementation and training of this pilot with your district's facilities and food service managers. Partnership does require you provide access to facilities for monthly pest monitoring, pest control records, and pilot school custodial/ kitchen staff for a one-time, one-to-two-hour training session. The staff training will be provided on-site and scheduled for your convenience.

I would like to congratulate you on becoming what I am confident will be a model school for this type of proactive management program. I do realize that your time is valuable and your "plate is overflowing". However, I would ask that you communicate your commitment to "test drive" this program with your custodial and kitchen staff, as well as your faculty. Please feel free to contact me regarding any questions regarding this program at (contact phone number and email address). Further, I believe that your district's administrator in Facilities Management can also provide insight regarding our partnership. I look forward to meeting you in the future and introducing you to my implementation team during our visit in January.

Sincerely,
Dr. Marc L. Lame

cc: (all pilot school principals and the district's facility and food service managers)

I try to limit these letters to one page, introduce myself as a fellow educator, describe what the IPM model is, who the implementers are, what they will provide and what I need from the principal. I always let them know I realize their plate is full and that they already are doing good things for their school community.

Once on board, principals usually are easy and even fun to work with. However, never forget that it is their gatekeeper — the principal's secretary —who really runs the school.. Fortunately, these wonderful folks have developed pretty good senses of humor and usually get a kick out of bug people.

During one of my recent programs I sent the December newsletter (containing District IPM update, Pantry Pests, Bobby's waste management tips) to our pilot schools. It was an outstanding letter, of course, EXCEPT that a story headline (in large bold type) read <u>Panty</u> Pests instead of Pantry Pests. OOPS. The high school principal's secretary called me on Friday explaining (between fairly lengthy interruptions of laughter) that they sent it out to all faculty and staff of the three schools. Teachers (notice I did not say university professors), being fairly good proofreaders, immediately began e-mailing the principal's office with some fairly humorous observations — fortunately. The secretary wanted me to catch the blunder in case I sent the newsletter out nationwide.

I apologized and explained that I was an entomologist, not a speller. Never have been. I asked her to e-mail the teachers back to let them know:

1) When I was a high school student I spent more time on the bench in front of the vice-principal's office than in class ;
2) that I appreciated their tolerance and humor;
3) that if any of them did have PANTY pests to please feel free to give me a call as I did have some experience regarding IPM and crab lice (take this as you will); and
4) that their vice principal and old friend from my teen years was responsible for proofreading. She and her faculty definitely enjoyed some comic relief at Dr. Lame's expense.

- **Custodial and Kitchen supervisors –**

Each school has a custodial and kitchen supervisor — sometimes the only staff person for that area, but a supervisor nonetheless. While these individuals have limited powers, they operate where the rubber meets the road. Within the confines of implementing real IPM, they work with the on-site IPM coordinator on cultural and mechanical control. If we expect schools to manage pests in partnership with a professional pest manager, we should empower these folks as full partners.

The best way to do this is by respecting them as professionals. They are, in fact, masters of their domain, and the majority of such people I have dealt with take professional pride in what they do for their school community. I learn their names and use Mr. or Ms. until they tell me otherwise. I learn from them their procedures for preparing meals and/or providing a sanitary space for their students and faculty. They have a lot to teach, and the best way to learn is to teach. It is relatively easy to relate their professional know-how to managing pests, and when you do that they become empowered.

Communicating with this audience is primarily a face-to-face proposition and works best when they are working. They get a little nervous if they are not getting their required chores done.

- **Public Relations (media flak)** –

If you want to spread the word for IPM, locally or nationally, you need a PR person — I affectionately call them "flaks". The real PR pros can very effectively market your message. That is their job. Public awareness of IPM in schools as an innovation and confirming that it works is critical for success and expansion. It is political management. I know one or two entomologists (and maybe a few school officials) who have some idea how PR works. I try to include a PR person when I can. Often they are employees of a state environmental agency or large school district. However, the best I work with are private sector folks like John Godec in Arizona, an old friend and colleague from my days with the Arizona Department of Environmental Quality. Fortunately, helping kids is often viewed as a reasonable pro-bono activity in this profession. John does it for the kids and usually scores some beer off me in the process.

PR pros can teach you how to capitalize on your success and save you lots of time and embarrassment. It is their job to know who to contact in the mass media (television, newspaper, radio, etc.) that might be looking for this type of story. Many of us bug types think IPM is the story — big mistake. Kids, pesticides and/or pest-related disease are the story. School districts saving money —or better yet, wasting money on inefficient pest control — is the story.

John taught me not to waste reporters' time, to help them write the story, meet their deadlines and to be fair about who gets the story first. These are basic ethics for media relations. He taught me to plan for media visits with the scariest scorpions posed for pictures, and parents ready to testify. Of course he also taught me to amuse myself with their professional quirks and gross-out factor when it came to rats and roaches.

These are essential resources you must manage if you want to change the world, but change is a process, and in the political world that process is called policymaking.

Chapter Thirteen – Policymaking for School IPM – "Talk is cheap"

IPM is a process, not a miracle. It requires nurturing and confirmation to keep going. The opportunity for IPM will always have to come in response to a call from you — the concerned school community member — but action should be complemented by those who have a mission to protect our health and environment. Providing a safe learning environment, what so many good people have worked so hard for, is "the right thing to do" for our children, ourselves, our professions and our planet. This specific environmental innovation — Integrated Pest Management — that I have outlined for you and tried to convince you to adopt, is highly effective. However, I do worry that the school systems I worked with will revert to pesticide dependence. It is happening already.

This book has presented a number of individual types and people who actually implement ("do") IPM. I have discussed how, "by doing", implementers can change a community by influencing diffusion of innovations like IPM. If an innovation has a relative advantage over an existing practice, is compatible with the community's norms, values and beliefs, and can be tried and observed then it can be sustained by the adopting community. However, do we provide job security and resources for implementers of IPM who attempt to change their community's behavior? How do we change the world in the context of pest management? In this final chapter I will discuss the most fundamental evolution of democratic social change – Policymaking. I will describe the pitfalls of policy as a Band-Aid® solution, and plead for you to TAKE CONTROL.

According to Colebatch: Policy is 1)"an idea which flows through all the ways in which we organize our life"; and 2) "a concept in the analysis of the process of government"; but also 3) "is part of the process which it describes" (Colebatch, 2002, p. vi). For the purposes of this chapter, I will define policy in terms of what it should do:

> **Policy** – provides guidelines for: 1) What action needs to be taken; 2) who should take that action; and 3) how to support those taking action. Good policy should result in successful implementation.

There is no national policy for government agencies to implement IPM in schools, other than as it may be convenient to protect and promote American agribusiness. Therefore there is no plan for real implementation, and for damn' sure, no funds earmarked to provide "a safe learning environment". The USDA has a "road map" that talks about IPM in schools. However, from what I have observed, that agency's "support" goes more toward studies. Cooperative Extension personnel who implement IPM in schools are seldom supported, let alone rewarded.

A more disturbing fact I will discuss in this chapter is that the USEPA has no policy for implementing IPM in our nation's schools, either. Several years ago I offered to help the USEPA develop a national policy and implementation plan for school IPM. This draft was, in part, a product of the graduate students in my capstone course on environmental policy. What the class found in the development of an implementation plan was that the USEPA did not know what it wanted in terms of IPM in schools, who should implement IPM in schools or what resources were needed (let alone being provided) to facilitate that implementation (Lame, et. al, 2001). The USEPA had great intentions, and dedicated staff, but little leadership. This *Draft Implementation Plan for Integrated Pest Management in Schools* provided the USEPA with strategies for implementing IPM in schools nationwide and, predictably, resulted in more discussion about what would it take for the adoption of this initiative/policy. No USEPA policy decision resulted from such discussion.

Whether by design or fiat, the USEPA in its zeal to partner with the USDA, Tribes and state lead agencies has cobbled together a cruise ship with loads of similar passenger activities but no rudder. In all fairness, while I work with several USEPA work groups that want to implement pesticide reduction programs to protect children, I am in no way privy to all their management decisions. It is quite possible the administration of this agency decided a long time ago that the best policy was no policy. In fact, this incremental approach to policymaking is not uncommon (Kingdon, 1995). However, just how long, or how many successful programs, does it take for this agency to provide a more aggressive directive? By not making any real policy decisions it has left the steering of the ship to co-opted and under-funded state agencies. Eighteen states have agencies with policies for IPM in schools. To my knowledge, not one of these has a fully funded mandate for implementation.

Do these federal and state agencies (that have, at least, an implied public mandate to provide a safe learning environment) provide some funding to implement IPM? Yes. Do they believe it is "the right thing to do"? I believe so — at least at ground level. As individuals, are many of these government officials willing to take risks to put IPM to work in our nation's child-sensitive facilities? Yes. So why are school systems not adopting IPM or, worse, reverting to pesticide dependence? Because the terms "some funding", believing it is "the right thing to do", and forcing unprotected faculty or government employees to take risks are not enough of themselves to change the national norm for pest management. Talk is cheap.

What about your school district policy for IPM? I know there are real, verifiable IPM programs in schools across our country. However, EVERY school district that I have approached with regard to IPM has stated, "We do IPM...we have a policy!" In the 10 years I have been implementing IPM in schools, NOT ONE was actually conducting a real IPM program but I will discuss that later.

Our Policy Decisionmakers -

Let us understand that our government works in two basic ways: talking and doing. Unless a national crisis looms, our elected officials rarely do anything but talk. Most voters really like this even if they say otherwise. "Status quo" perpetuates predictable economic and political outcomes, stability and bureaucratic constipation. It is comfortable (well, maybe not the constipation thing). Change is unpredictable, risky, labor intensive and uncomfortable. In fact, when it comes to lobbyists and policymaking, most lobbyist activities revolve around blocking new policies or changes to existing policies. Most money for lobbyists is spent maintaining the status quo.

I suggest, to those of you who want to change the world to work both ends of the street — get the right talk and assure that it gets implemented. Understand what it takes to get politicians and bureaucrats (who are supposed to protect our children's health and the environment) to do their jobs. Both talkers and doers in government live in a world of problems they aspire to fix. Whether it is the existing policies (funded, under-funded and unfunded) that address those problems or the political decisions that govern whether those policies are successfully implemented depends on who is forcing decisionmakers to do their job. "Who" is you — there is need for active participants at all levels of government.

Who "does" policy?

What does an entomologist know about policy? Nothing. On the other hand, what do policymakers know about entomology? Ever heard of Africanized Bees (a.k.a., Killer Bees)? Leon Moore once told me (Moore, 1991) he had a hard time getting an article published because of policy. Leon wrote that Africanized Bees would cross the border from Mexico to Arizona sometime in the early 1990s. He was told he couldn't write that in a government publication because the position of the USDA was that these insects wouldn't arrive in our country that soon. Sure enough, the bees were in town by 1992.

We entomologists look at our bugs (what a great life — sex, bugs and rock 'n' roll). Unfortunately, we are weak on program, resource and political management and just plain ignorant regarding how our programs are created, funded and maintained. Some learn by doing, many just founder, pigs at the trough who squeal when poked. As you read in chapter four, my ignorance cost me my career as an Extension entomologist. However, that experience played a major influence in my graduate learning experience.

In the mid-1980s and about five frustrating years into attempting to implement IPM with Arizona cotton farmers, I decided to earn another degree while working full-time as an entomologist for the University of Arizona. I was really curious regarding what it took for communities to adopt innovations. As it turned out, this course of study fell under the School of Public Administration at Arizona State University. I was directed to two scholars in charge of the program at the time, Louis Weschler and L. A. Wilson. They convinced me that another degree would indeed further my education and satisfy my intellectual curiosity.

Seven, part-time years later I had another degree. Now, I do not recommend this path of enlightenment. Being of average intelligence I was in too deep before I knew I was a masochist — not to mention a rube. Lou and L.A. were both avid fly fishermen and were willing to say anything to entice an entomologist (someone to identify trout "flies") to become one of their graduate students.

A Ph.D. in Public Administration allows the holder to study the theory and practice of how public agencies are managed and how they can work better. Not only did I learn about the diffusion of innovation but also about public finance, public personnel management, loads of statistics, public program evaluation and public policy. I hated the way my professors wanted me to learn. It was not at all like becoming a learned entomologist. Instead of requiring students to memorizing organisms, their biology, chemistry associated with living organisms and methods for observing and studying these organisms, Public Administration is a social science that requires elaborate discussion of each topic. This meant, after years of concise "just the facts, ma'am" written material, I was expected to write lengthy observations of paradigms, contexts and concepts. Weird stuff. However, after a year or two of Lou and L.A. propping me up (while I taught them about which insects were about to emerge for catching the most trout) the light did come on.

There was a whole world out there that spoke a different language and marched to a different beat than that spoken and marched to by hard scientists, and it ruled! I learned that for my program (in this case, implementing IPM in cotton) to work I had to understand the intent of the program, what resources were needed to make it work, and how to obtain those resources. That is political management. Insects? Hmmph. Humans just think we manage them. I finally understood that pest management is people management.

I have discussed what actions must be taken to protect our children from pests and pesticides in our schools and who should take that action. Understanding the public policy behind IPM in schools gave me a better idea of how to manage the what and who, but more importantly it opened my eyes how to obtain the resources to make it happen.

Public Policy for School IPM 101

Much of how I explain the making of public policy comes from a text I use when teaching the policy process — *Agendas, Alternatives, and Public Policies* by John W. Kingdon. I know just enough about policymaking to be dangerous. So bear with me. Public policymaking in our system is composed of four fundamental parts: Setting the agenda, choosing an alternative, authorizing a specific alternative and implementing that alternative (Kingdon, 1995).

The Agenda addresses the problem that our school community (primarily children) lacks a safe learning environment because of inadequate pest management and unreasonable exposure caused by unnecessary use of pesticides. Spillover of other real or perceived problems in the school community — lack of school funding and concern about indoor air quality — could affect this agenda. School districts are always particularly sensitive to the economic and political consequences of complying with federal mandates for student achievement and student safety.

The Alternatives to address this problem are numerous:

- the pesticide industry pushes the "no change, current or traditional" model of "spray and pray";
- (probably the most pervasive) changing the name of exterminator to pest control operator or technician and telling everyone you practice IPM, but don't, and charge schools more;
- the technical smorgasbord of partial IPM offered by some Pest Management Professionals that does not mandate full participation of the school district — it's technically IPM but out of sight/out of mind for the lazy school administrator;
- the we-won't-use-any-pesticide-ever model championed by the well-meaning anti-pesticide folks; and
- real IPM in partnership with an educated, participating school district.

These all are possible alternatives. The alternative that becomes authorized by decisionmakers depends on how those decisionmakers are lobbied:

- who the "policy entrepreneurs" are and their abilities;
- which alternative is more technically feasible and socially acceptable; and
- which alternative can anticipate and/or overcome significant constraints (Kingdon, 1995).

However, the best alternative might not see the light of day unless a plethora of stars align.

Kingdon describes three major process streams that must "couple" when setting the agenda and changing policy:

1. Problem recognition or "Problem Stream" in which problems capture the attention of decisionmakers;
2. formation or refinement of policy proposals – "Policy Stream" - where solutions (alternatives) to problems are developed; and
3. "Political Stream" in which factors such as public opinion, national mood and changes of administration allow for the notice of alternatives (Kingdon, 1995).

"The separate streams come together at critical times. A problem is recognized, a solution is available, the political climate makes the time right for change, and the constraints do not prohibit action" (Kingdon, p. 88). These streams converge or couple through the proverbial window of opportunity when a new policy is ready to be implemented. It is like giving birth, and the parents who join together and nurture their embryo to meet the challenges of the cold cruel world are called policy entrepreneurs.

As you might imagine, a great deal of yelling, moaning and screaming is associated with bringing this baby policy into the world. It is not a pretty sight, but if done correctly, can produce beautiful outcomes. So I have tried to develop my strategy for policy entrepreneurship as it pertains to IPM in schools by determining answers to the following questions:

- Do decisionmakers at local, state or federal levels even recognize that "the school community (primarily children) lacks a safe learning environment because of inadequate pest management and unreasonable exposure to unnecessary use of pesticides"?

No- Decisionmakers at local, state and national levels seldom think about a safe learning environment in terms other than drugs and violence. As I mentioned at the beginning of this book, school administrators are barraged with under- or unfunded mandates on nearly any conceivable topic. Sometimes these topics relate to school safety. Of late the hot topic is accountability, otherwise known as testing. Pest management is not on their radar screen until TV cameras arrive to tape footage of rats, there is a disease outbreak related to pests, or children are evacuated due to pesticide exposure. Elected officials at all levels are even further removed. However, some state agency administrators who occasionally champion children's environmental health would like to elevate the awareness of IPM. Of course, the USEPA mid-level folks are keen on implementing IPM, but they are subject to the political aspirations of the current Administrator (appointed by the President) — just another decisionmaker whose radar screen does not register pests and pesticide exposure in schools as a problem.

- Is "real IPM in partnership with an educated, participating school district" (the most technically feasible, socially acceptable alternative that has the ability to anticipate and/or overcome significant constraints) been made available to decisionmakers?

Yes - It is well demonstrated and documented that IPM as we implement it in schools is not only technically feasible, but also highly effective in reducing pests without increasing costs. It is socially acceptable because of its cost effectiveness, but also because it most closely approaches what the public wants with regard to its children's learning environment — that is, no pests, no pesticides. If implemented correctly in schools, IPM overcomes the major constraints of increasing costs and "adding more to their plate" that so many members of the school community fear and hate. By demonstrating their participation in the IPM partnership they can "do what they are doing now", in terms of education, sanitation, energy management and security, but "just think pests".

- Does the public and its administrators (school superintendents, state lead agency directors, the USEPA, Congress and the President) have the desire or are they in the mood to address this problem with this solution?

Maybe – If the window of opportunity for policy formulation is open, decisionmakers might just jump through it. Some of the public and some administrators (school superintendents, state lead agency directors, the USEPA, Congress and the President) have the desire and are in the mood to change the status quo and address the fact that school communities lack a safe learning environment. It has become a national scandal that schools have to do more with less. IPM, as I have described it, more effectively manages pests with less (pesticides and, normally, money). The public is beginning to understand that what we allow in our schools in terms of food and chemicals can have detrimental effects on our children's ability to learn. The public is coming to no longer believe that drug or pesticide manufacturers are working in their best interests. Last, in the wake of the unfunded "no child left behind" mandate, both the public and its administrators are now more aware that feel-good legislation without adequate funding is ruining our public school system.

Whether decisionmakers jump through this window of opportunity depends on whether you push them and just how you push them. Well, I am pushing by writing this book. There are other ways to push, but first let me discuss how a few IPM–in–schools policies are creating obstacles to reaching the goal of verifiable, sustainable and profitable implementation.

Policies are nice – so what?

Talk is cheap. These days, every school district and almost every state I work in has an IPM policy. The IPM policy is critical for a sustainable program in each school district. However, if that policy is not monitored and enforced it is just cheap talk that turned into paper.

The Monroe IPM Model was developed in Indiana almost 10 years ago. One might assume that this state would have fully implemented IPM in its nearly 300 school districts by now. It has not happened. In my opinion it is because the change agents in Indiana relied on policymaking, rather than implementation, to do their job for them. In 1999, the Indiana Pesticide Review Board drafted a policy that allowed all Indiana school districts to voluntarily adopt IPM. The policy offered the help of numerous stakeholders, including Improving Kids' Environment director Tom Neltner. Below is Tom's (Improving Kids' Environment Newsletter, 2000) summary of that policy:

> **Training:** If staff of a school district applies pesticides, the district must have a certified pesticide applicator supervise the staff and staff must receive annual training. Currently, no training is required beyond federal hazard communication required by OSHA.
>
> **Prohibited Uses:** Unless the label is more restrictive, no pesticides may be applied in the presence of children. Pesticides that leave a residue on exposed surfaces or could become airborne may only be used from two hours before school begins until one hour after school ends where the pests pose an immediate threat or a serious disruption.
>
> **Advance Notice:** Parents, teachers, and staff will be asked whether they want to receive advance notice of pesticide use. Health professionals in the school will receive notice automatically. Those who request notice should be notified by the school at least two days in advance of the pesticide use. If advance notice is not provided, the school needs to explain the delay and what pesticides were used.
> The advance notice must include:
>
> - Anticipated date of pesticide use;
> - General location of pesticide use; and
> - Phone number to call for more information.
>
> If pesticides might be applied during a routine scheduled service inspection, rather than encourage a long listing of all potential pesticides, the school can provide the results of the last service inspection.

Access to Records: Schools must make available details of the pests encountered and pesticides used for 90 days from the application.

Exemptions:

- Pesticides used in normal cleaning activities;
- Personal insect repellents when self-applied;
- Human or animal ectoparasite control products (primarily to deal with lice) administered by a professional;
- Manufactured enclosed, paste or gel bait insecticides where students do not have access to bait.

In my opinion, this is an excellent policy for pesticide reduction. However, it does not address the implementation of IPM other than to provide incentives for alternate pest management techniques, thereby eliminating the need to notify the parents regarding pesticide use. To my knowledge, fewer than five school districts in Indiana actually are implementing verifiable IPM programs.

In late 2004 the Pesticide Review Board met to discuss the status of IPM in schools. Based on the "inspections" of a State Lead Agency employee, 29 of 40 schools were described as having had adopted an IPM policy. Reasons given by school officials for not adopting an IPM policy were under-staffing, no funds and not understanding the IPM policy". It was decided that the State Lead Agency should continue to conduct inspections at schools, and consider surveying school district participation (Indiana Pesticide Review Board minutes -November, 2004).

It would be interesting to know what is meant by the term "inspection". Adopting a policy is far different than implementing a policy — with all abundant respect due our elected officials. It is my experience, as I work to implement IPM in schools nationwide, that most states with IPM policies (in law, rule or agreement) have a dismal implementation rate. We can only hope the criteria for adoption include implementation. One sure way to ascertain whether significant implementation is occurring in the 29 schools that have "passed" inspection is to subject them to something like Tom Green's IPM Star® program (IPM Institute of North America).

I recollect that a survey of Indiana school districts conducted several years ago by the IPM Technical Resource Center at Purdue University pegged the adoption rate at more than 90% (Fournier, 2002). These results are identical to the IPM policy adoption rate in Florida school districts. For a number of years, the Florida Department of Education (Althouse, Personal Conversation, 2004) conducted surveys of schools adopting and implementing IPM. They achieved significant numbers — over 90%. Upon questioning however, all state agency surveyors and University of Florida entomologists agreed that implementation was actually less than 10% (Oi, Personal Conversation, 2004) I am currently working with the University of Florida's number one pick for an implementing school district, Brevard Public Schools. It turns out they were implementing a bait substitution program, not IPM (to the standards agreed on by our team), but thanks to a very professional and committed administration are now preparing for the IPM Star® certification. They just did not have or utilize a model of what IPM was supposed to be.

In short, further surveys or "inspections" of IPM policy implementation without verification invite false positives. It is not surprising that four years after approving a voluntary, unfunded policy focused on pesticide reduction instead of IPM implementation, Indiana school districts did not implement IPM. They did not know what IPM was (what action to take), were under-staffed (who was to take this action) and unfunded (lacked the resources to take action). Nice policy, but bad targeting.

My change agent friends in Indiana did attempt a diffusion process, but halfheartedly followed through in the implementation and confirmation stages. I suspect it was just too easy to rely on the old "give 'em facts sheets, manuals, workshops and an 'information hotline'" model of diffusion. This model is called the Hypodermic Needle Model because change agents merely inject the community with information about the supposed innovation (Katz, 1957). Worse, these policies were crafted under pressure from the school district administrator and pest control industry lobbyists to delay implementation of IPM until the concerned public yawned and moved on to other issues. Typically, Cooperative Extension and the state pesticide regulatory agency responded with informational tools and requests to "study" the situation further. Yeah, I am a bit jaded by now.

You might be asking: why has Indiana failed to fully implement IPM if Marc Lame patrolled its skies in his superhero tights? I tried for a while, but I had the opportunity to work with school districts and change agents elsewhere who really felt a strong need or were empowered to "do the right thing". It also taught me that sometimes you just have to move on and let friends do their own thing.

Strategies of this "policy entrepreneur":

Please know I hate the word entrepreneur, especially when describing myself. I don't cater to French-sounding words, the "e" word is too often associated with business schools and it sounds like "manure". My strategies are multifaceted and based on two fundamentals: Follow Ev Roger's Innovation-Decision process and do what I do best — demonstrate IPM. These strategies are meant to address the answers to "coupling" (see Public Policy for School IPM 101): Decisionmakers are not aware of the need for IPM in schools, that IPM in schools is technically feasible and socially acceptable, and that the public just might be in the mood to change the way school districts protect our school children from pests and pesticides.

Demonstrate – prove it! What I try to demonstrate to the school community, the public and policymakers with the Monroe IPM Model and its team of implementers is that IPM has undeniable positive attributes and can easily overcome the pain of change:

- The relative advantage of IPM over traditional "exterminator" models of pest management in terms of effectiveness, cost and safety;
- the compatibility of IPM with the school community's culture as it addresses educational value, support function integration (sanitation, maintenance and administration) — "do what you are doing now, just think pests";
- that the school community can try IPM in pilot schools without a total commitment;
- that the school community can observe the results of IPM in terms of fewer pest complaints, applications of pesticides and appreciation of community members, change agents and peer school systems; and
- the complexity of the IPM innovation is mitigated by the existing safety, energy management and security requirements already practiced in well-managed school districts.

Demonstrating IPM in schools this way raises the level of awareness in our policymakers that the "exterminator" model of pest management is a problem in terms of safety and cost. It proves that IPM is a technically feasible facility management paradigm and is accepted by school social systems. It does help create a mood in the public that this change in management is both needed and doable.

Transfer it – make sense beyond the schools. Perhaps in this last task of mood change we all could do better. While my world might revolve around IPM, maybe there is a better way to relate to the public. "Spillover" is a policymaking term that essentially means we need to "look outside our box". Here, then, the philosophy of IPM as practiced by most implementers (sometimes including me) has been too narrowly focused in the context of folks who work for our schools and entomology. I suspect the political base for IPM could be expanded by promoting IPM education to the public specific to school and home pest management, but with regard to a general awareness of public health and environmental concerns that could be adopted by all pesticide users (municipalities, our workplace, community centers, elderly and childcare, etc.).

Market it – creating partnerships with the passionate and the capitalists. Management of public programs increasingly goes beyond mandates to marketing. Thus I use the Innovation-Decision process to push the public and our decisionmakers through the IPM window of opportunity. However, this is not a one-man show. Those responsible for policy decisions (children's health advocates, government regulators, school officials, professional pest managers, etc.), program development and program implementation concerning pesticide use and pest management would do well to consider the importance of communication as a management skill. But they also need to incorporate the sub-specialty of diffusion in their strategic communication plans. This is why I choose to influence my fellow entomologists, pest management professionals and government regulators into becoming better change agents. And, even more daunting, work with school business officials and the pest control industry to develop a business model that is verifiable, sustainable and profitable.

In this book I have mentioned that most professionals who work with me, sustain me, lead me and follow me have certain traits. All want to "do the right thing" for our school children, some revert to a child-like delight when playing with bugs, some enjoy a good fight, some just want to finally do what they thought they were hired to do. However, those who have become my partners have more — passion. My definition of passion is not simply fervent enthusiasm but *needing* beyond what is physically and emotionally expected. Thus IPM, as I practice and define it, is an innovation that meets the needs of this passionate community as well, and therefore my use of the Innovation-Decision process to diffuse the Monroe IPM Model by this community of change agents. In this process, my friends, colleagues and partners in "changing the world" have not only adopted this model, they have reinvented it and become owners of it as well (Rice and Rogers, 1980, Lame, 1997). I do recognize that we must provide job security and resources to these change agents. This battle continues and I ask the reader to assist these passionate ones, who put themselves at professional risk, as well.

Well, I guess making a profit can be a passion. I figure it is just a way of life for most folks in our society. Please don't fool yourself that university faculty don't want to make a profit. Unfortunately, I have worked with some who seem to have profit making as their prime motivation. Money never has meant much to me other than to provide for my family, buying some fun toys, beer for my friends, and changing the world. However, if you want to motivate industry, you have to do it with profit extended as a carrot.

It is my opinion that school districts should internalize the pest management function just as they do with indoor air quality, energy management and security functions. I have discussed the reasons for this in this book in terms of providing better communication, organizational management and more cost efficiency. However, in my experience, school districts with fewer than 15 schools find it difficult to employ a pest management professional. Thus, many larger school districts will want to use an outside contractor, and most small districts will need to contract with a pest control company. Procurement of services becomes the name of the game (Greene and Breisch, 2002). Know with certainty, as mentioned in chapter three, this relationship MUST BE A PARTNERSHIP! Not an out-of-sight, out-of-mind contractual function. Given that almost all of pest management in schools is cultural control (not attracting pests) and mechanical control (excluding pests) the school community should provide the vast majority of pest management for its facilities. However, each school district must utilize a pest management professional to diagnose and educate.

The question to which I have not ascertained an answer to is, how can the pest control industry become a partner with the school district, provide a sustainable, verifiable IPM program and still make a profit? I am currently trying to develop a business plan with schools and this industry to answer that question. The short and simple answer is that the school district business official who understands what real IPM is and what a real pest management professional should provide must then determine:

- What portion of pest management is the school community's responsibility?
- How much time should the pest management professional spend in each school annually to diagnose pest infestations and conducive conditions (via written documentation)?
- How much time should the pest management professional spend educating appropriate staff to identify pests, document pests, recognize conducive conditions and remediate conducive conditions?

- How much time will the pest management professional need to occasionally eliminate a pest infestation?

These procurement protocols sound simple enough but require some very soul-searching answers from both partners. The facts is that I am still trying to develop a trusting relationship with school districts and the pest control industry so I can answer those questions. School officials are hesitant to admit they don't know what pest management really costs their school district. For instance, I have never talked to a school business official that understood the industry charges $60 per hour (Martin, Personal Conversation, 2005) Most contractual bids are based on per school or per square foot rate, and the business officials (or procurement officers) have no idea how much time actually is required for management professionals to do their job. As I have studied contracts with Carl Martin and John Carter, I sometimes feel as though I am trying to decide what car lease agreement I should sign. These agreements seem comprised of smoke and mirrors. Without doubt, pest control industry managers understand that this partnership will require genuine accountability, not to mention a reduction in revenue, as school districts become better trained at handling the majority of their pest management chores (and becoming less pesticide-dependent in the process). I suspect if we ever do develop these answers, school districts that contract with pest control companies will probably need to have a flexible long-term payment schedule that would decline over time. Am I trying to create a trusting relationship with the pest control industry? Yes, but I doubt this book, my final strategic weapon, will induce the pest control industry to grow warm, fuzzy and trusting about climbing into bed with Marc Lame.

Conclusion

Join the battle and provide the ammo – write the book.

I wrote this book as a means to convince our decisionmakers they need to adopt and support IPM as a means of protecting our schoolchildren. It is a broad strategy that I always knew must one day be employed. Because scientists can use their language and write for their peers, it is relatively straightforward to write articles for peer-reviewed and sometimes obscure journals. Writing a book for public consumption is an entirely different proposition, although I have to admit it is somewhat pleasurable to write as I normally speak — instead of as a professorial prig. That fact combined with the reality that I would rather work (and play) "in the field" with those as passionate as I regarding protecting children and the environment, has allowed me to delay writing this book. Several decent published manuals

207

provide directions for managing pests in schools via IPM. However, as one who wants to drive policy at local, state and national levels, I know that those who want to change the world when it comes to their school community's health need a readable text that provides directions for effectively managing people in order to achieve better pest management. "Pest management is people management".

At this point I imagine you understand that IPM has opponents and proponents. It is time to provide those who want a healthier school community with the ammunition to refute decades-old propaganda from those who would rather sell you pesticides (or a service to expose your children to them) month after month. I hope I have entertained you at times by writing colloquially and expressing my true love of entomology. More importantly, I hope I have communicated as I intended by providing information to help you protect our children from pests and pesticides in their schools, perhaps influenced your behavior and affected your attitudes about what rational pest management in truth should be. It is my sincere hope that this text will stimulate diffusion of IPM in the national school community, and just maybe, increase diffusion of IPM in our homes, workplaces and agricultural communities. I have begun the process of change — now it's your turn.

References

Althouse, E. (2003). Personal Conversation. Informal Scoping Session on School IPM Certification for Florida. University of Florida. February 20, 2004

Anonymous, (2004). Personal and Confidential Communication with nationally known urban entomologist and Marc L. Lame.

Avery, D. T. (2000). *Saving the Planet with Pesticides and Plastic.* Indianapolis, IN: Hudson Institute.

Basso, C. J. (1987). *Pesticides and Politics.* Pittsburgh: University of Pittsburgh Press.

Bennett, G., Owens, J. and Corrigan, R (2003). *Truman's Scientific Guide to Pest Management Operations* (6th ed.). Cleveland: Advanstar Communications.

Berenbaum, M. R. (1995). *Bugs in the System: Insects and Their Impact on Human Affairs.* New York: Addison-Wesley

Bourgoin, C. (2003). Personal Conversation.

Braband, Horn & Sahr (2002). *Pest Management Practices: A survey of public school districts in New York State.* NYS IPM Program, NYSAES, Geneva, NY. NYS IPM Number 613.

Carson, R. (1962). *Silent Spring* (1st ed.). Boston: Houghton-Mifflin.

Cline, H. (2001), "School anti-pesticide drive is everyone's fight in nation". *Western Farm Press* (November 3, 2001).

Colebatch, H. K. (2002). *Policy* (2nd ed.). Buckingham, U.K.: Open University Press.

Congress of the United States, House of Representatives, (2002). Letter from Mr. Jay Vroom and Mr. Allen James to EOA Assistant Administrator Stephen L. Johnson (July 8, 2002).

Congress of the United States, House of Representatives, (2002). Letter from EPA Assistant Administrator Stephen L. Johnson to Mr. Jay Vroom (August, 2002).

Corrigan, R. M. (2001). *Rodent Control: A Practical Guide for Pest Management Professionals.* Cleveland: GIE Media.

Debrewer, L. and Hokanson, D. (1996). *Adopting Integrated Pest Management in the Monroe County Community School Corporation: Case Study and Analysis.* Unpublished report to the MCCSC School Board, Bloomington, IN.

Disraeli, B (1804 -1881). Quotation #487 from Michael Moncur's (Cynical) Quotations (1985).

Downs, G.W., Jr. & Mohr, L.B. *Toward a Theory of Innovation.* (Discussion Paper 92). Ann Arbor: University of Michigan, Institute of Public Policy Studies.

Eskenazi, B., Bradman, A. and Castorina, R. (1999). Exposures of children to organophosphate pesticides and their potential adverse health effects. *Environmental Health Perspectives* 107 (Suppl. 3):409-19.

Fournier, A. (2002). "Update on Indiana School IPM", 2002 Purdue Pest Control Conference, West Lafayette, Indiana.

Garnett, J. L. (1992). *Communicating for Results in Government: A Strategic Approach for Public Managers.* San Francisco, Jossey-Bass publishers.

Geier, P. W. (1966). Management of Insect Pests. *Ann. Rev. Entomol.* 11: 471-490.

Goldman, L. R. (1995). Children—unique and vulnerable: environmental risks facing children and recommendations for response. *Environmental Health Perspectives* 103 (Suppl. 6):13-18.

Gouge, D. H., Stoltman, A. J., Snyder, J. L. and Olson, C. (2004). *How to Bug Proof Your Home.* Tucson: The University of Arizona, Cooperative Extension (AZ1320).

Graham, L. C. (2001). Personal Conversation.

Greene, A. and Breisch, N (2002). Measuring Integrated Pest Management Programs for Public Buildings. *Journal of Economic Entomology*, 95, (1): 1-13.

Hokanson, D. and Debrewer, L. (1995). *Pest Management Analysis and Policy Recommendations: A Report to the Monroe County Community School Corporation.* Unpublished report to the MCCSC School Board, Bloomington, IN.

Indiana Pesticide Review Board (1999). "Recommendations for Pest Control by School Districts". I.P.R.B. minutes, December, 1999.

Katz, E. (1957). The Two-Step Flow of Communication: An Up-To-Date Report on a Hypothesis. *Public Opinions Quarterly*, 21, 61-78.

Kingdon, J. W. (1995). *Agendas, Alternatives, and Public Policies*, (2nd ed.) New York: Addison-Wesley Educational Publishers Inc.

Kubista-Hovis, K. & Lame, M. L. (2004). "The Economics of School Integrated Pest Management: An Analysis of th Monroe IPM Model in Bloomington, Indiana. *National Schools Update.* USEPA, BPPD, 1, (3): 5-7.

Lambur, M. T., Whalon, M. E. & Fear, F. A. (1985). Diffusion Theory and Integrated Pest Management: Illustrations from the Michigan Fruit IPM Program. *Bulletin of the Entomological Society of America*, 31, (2): 40-45.

Lame, M. L. (2001). *Extension of a Successful IPM Model to Pilot School Districts in States Currently Not Practicing IPM in Public Schools.* USEPA Pesticide Environmental Stewardship Partnership Grant Final Narrative Report.

Lame, M. L. (1999). *Extension of a Successful IPM Model to Pilot School Districts in States Currently Not Practicing IPM in Public Schools.* USEPA Pesticide Environmental Stewardship Partnership Grant Proposal.

Lame, M. L. (1997). Communicating in the Innovation Process: Issues and Guidelines (187-201), *Handbook of Administrative Communication* (Garnett and Kouzmin editors), New York: Marcel Dekker, Inc.

Lame, M. L. (1992). *A Study of the Diffusion of Integrated Pest Management in a Cotton Growing Community.* Ph.D. Dissertation, Tempe, Arizona State University.

Lame, M. & Moore, L. (1989). An Integrated Pest Management Program for the Boll Weevil (*Anthonomus grandis*), in Central Arizona. *Proceedings of the Beltwide Cotton Production Research Conference*, 1, 248-249.

Lame, M. L. (1988). *How to Influence Arizona Agricultural Producers to adopt new technologies: A Case History of the Diffusion of Integrated Pest Management (IPM) with Arizona Cotton Growers.* Paper presented at the meeting of the International Communications Association, New Orleans, LA.

Lowy, J. (2005). "U. S. Lawn Care Industry Fighting back Against Pesticide Bans". Scripps Howard News Service.

Lumish, T. & Lame, M. (1999). *Economic Analysis of Integrated Pest Management in Schools and Childcare Facilities.* Unpublished Graduate Research Project, Indiana University, School of Public and Environmental Affairs.

Martin, C. (2005). Personal Communication.

Mattes, K. (1989). "Kicking the Pesticide Habit". *The Amicus Journal* (Fall 1989, p. 10-17).

Metcalf, R. L. and Luckmann, W. (1994). *Introduction to Insect Pest Management* (3rd ed.) New York: John Wiley & Sons, Inc.

Moore, L. (1991). Personal Conversation. Tucson, Arizona.

Neltner, T. (2000). *Indiana Schools: Reducing Exposure to Pests and Pesticides.* Improving Kids' Environment Newsletter, 2000 Edition

Odum, E. P. (1971). *Fundamentals of Ecology* (3rd ed.). Philadelphia: W. B. Saunders Co.

Oi, F. (2003). Personal Conversation. Informal Scoping Session on School IPM Certification for Florida University of Florida. February 20, 2004

O'Leary, R. (1994). The Bureaucratic Politic Paradox: The Case of Wetlands Legislation in Nevada. *Journal of Public Administration Research and Theory* 4:4, 443-467.

O'Leary, R., Durant, R. F., Fiorino, D. J. & Weiland, P. S. (1999). *Managing for the Environment: Understanding the Legal, Organizational, and Policy Challenges.* San Francisco: Jossey-Bass Inc.

Pimentel, D. (1997), *Techniques for Reducing Pesticide Use: Economic and Environmental Benefits.* New York: Wiley, John & Sons, Inc.

Perl, P. (2001), "Absolute Truth", The Washington Post. (May 13, 2001, p. W12)

Preuss, R. (2003), "Green cleaning champion takes on Rush Limbaugh", *Cleaning and Maintenance Management* (December 4, 2003).

Responsible Industry for a Sound Environment® (2002), "Integrated Pest Management: What It Is, How It Works, and Why Pesticides Must Remain an Option". RISE Fact Sheet.

Responsible Industry for a Sound Environment® (2002), "Why School Pesticide Bans Would Compromise Children's Health: 'All or Nothing' Positions Miss the Point – Use Pesticides Judiciously, But Have Them Available When Needed". RISE® Fact Sheet.

Responsible Industry for a Sound Environment® (2002), "Pesticides Used In Schools: Thoroughly Tested, Well-Regulated and Safely Used". RISE® Fact Sheet.

Responsible Industry for a Sound Environment® (2002), "New Threats and Ancient Foes: How Pests Threaten the Health of Children and the Public". RISE® Fact Sheet.

Responsible Industry for a Sound Environment® (1998), "Response to argument raised by the Zahm and Ward article, 'Pesticides and Cancer'". RISE® February 3, 1998.

Rice, R. E. & Rogers, E. M. (1980). Reinvention in the Innovation Process. *Knowledge: Creation, Diffusion, Utilization*, 1, 499-514.

Rogers, E. M. (1995). *Diffusion of Innovations*. (4th ed.) New York: The Free Press.

Rogers, E. M. & Shoemaker, F. F. (1971). *Communications of Innovations: A Cross Cultural Approach*. New York: The Free Press.

Rogers, E. M. & Kincaid, D. L. (1981). *Communication Networks: Toward a New Paradigm for Research*. New York: The Free Press.

Starling, G. (1993). *Managing the Public Sector*. (4th ed.) Belmont, CA, Wadsworth Publishing Co.

School of Public and Environmental Affairs, Indiana University, Graduate Capstone Class – Andersen, E., Andriyevska, L., Beekman, C., Burns, R., Crowley, K., Fox, J., Henry, D., Jackson, D., Lanier, D., McDavid, M., Park, H., Patti, N., Quirindongo, M., Riley, B., Roberts, B., Senne, P., Tsukada, H., and Weston, D. (2001). *Draft Implementation Plan for Integrated Pest Management in Schools* (under the direction of Marc L. Lame). Bloomington, Indiana.

United States Department of Agriculture (2001). "A National Road Map for Pest Management 2001-2010". USDA draft August, 15, 2001.

United States Environmental Protection Agency (1993). *Pest Control in the School Environment: Adopting Integrated Pest Management*. EPA 735-F-93-012. Washington, D.C.

United States Government Accounting Offices (1999). Pesticides – Use, Effects, and Alternatives to Pesticides in Schools, *GAO/RCED-00-17*

United States Government Accounting Offices (2001). Agricultural Pesticides - Management Improvements Needed to Further Promote Integrated Pest Management, *GAO-01-815*

Van Den Bosch, R. (1978). *The Pesticide Conspiracy.* Garden City, New York: Doubleday.

Ware, G., Moore, L. and Thrall, B. (1994). The University of Arizona College of Agriculture (recollections of from George Ware), The Arizona Historical Society, Oral History Programs (April 18, 1994).

Wearing, C. H. (1988). Evaluating The IPM Implementation Process. *Annual Review of Entomology,* 33, 17-38.

Wilson, E. O. (1987). "The Little Things That Run the World" from an address given at the opening of the invertebrate exhibit, National Zoological Park, Washington, D.C. *Conservation Biology,* 1, (4), 344-346.

Zahm, S. H. and Devesa S. S. (1995). Childhood cancer: overview of incidence trends and environmental carcinogens. *Environmental Health Perspectives* 103 (Suppl. 6):177-184.

Appendices

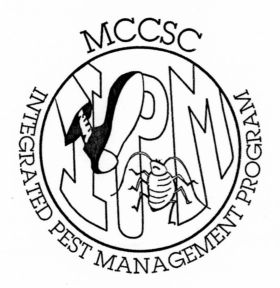

A.   What is Integrated Pest Management, and What is NOT Integrated Pest Management:

A reality check for school administrators considering the adoption of IPM
Marc L. Lame – Entomologist

Integrated Pest Management (IPM) DEFINED AS AN INNOVATION TO BE ADOPTED:
• IPM is a cluster of technologies (cultural, mechanical, biological, genetic, and chemical) which is an integrated application (based on biological information) designed to allow humans to compete with other species (pests).

Pest management in the school environment must be safe, and it should be cost effective. It has been widely documented that schools can significantly decrease risks to their inhabitants (students, faculty and staff) from pests and pesticides by implementing IPM. Further, that the implementation of IPM does not have to cost more than more traditional "extermination" programs. The IPM approach can be successful in the school environment because cultural (practices to reduce attracting pests) and mechanical strategies (practices to exclude pests) can be incorporated into the existing custodial and maintenance activities such as sanitation, energy conservation, building security and infrastructure maintenance. Monitoring efficiency (verification of pest presence) is enhanced via the virtual full time presence and perception of the school inhabitants. This strategy is dependent on an educational approach, which would create an awareness of all occupants on a proactive management strategy versus the reactive strategy of chemical treatment. Thus, by incorporating IPM into existing school operations (sanitation, maintenance, and classroom education) and "partnering" with a qualified Pest Management Professional as a consultant/educator (rather than as an "exterminator"), school districts will be able to overcome their natural resistance to "adding pest management to an already full plate".
IPM is:
- A management strategy based on communication/education which is supported by a committed school administration
- A "partnership" with the school community (including

219

concerned parents) and a qualified (i.e., the ability to technically apply and COMMUNICATE IPM) Pest Management Professional

- An educational system which empowers the school inhabitants to eliminate or reduce the reasons for insects, rodents and plants to become pests
- An educational system which empowers the school inhabitants to prevent pest from entering the school facility
- An educational system which empowers the school staff to know when to remedy and how to remedy documented pest problems by integrating cultural, mechanical and lowest impact chemical control technologies

IPM is NOT:

- A term or job description added to an unwilling or unqualified individual (the school district must either employ or contract with a qualified Pest Management Professional).
- A "low bid" process subject to unqualified exterminators, or qualified Pest Management Professionals who will not be able to perform to professional standards
- An "out of sight, out of mind" contractual function. The school community must be willing to communicate with their Pest Management Professional in order to facilitate long term cultural controls (practices to reduce attracting pests) and mechanical control (practices to exclude pests)
- A chemical pesticide program to prevent pests from entering schools
- A no chemical pesticide option. There are situations where chemical pesticides are necessary and can be used safely.

Professional educators know that communication/education is required to influence behavior. Influencing those whose behaviors allow pest problems to continue or occur in school is required for the successful implementation of IPM. Drawing back on my first years in graduate school I learned that first and foremost - "Insects (pests) can be managed, but management is people-oriented, and successful pest management depends largely on influencing the people who control the pest." (Metcalf and Luckmann, 1975).

B. Arizona IPM in Schools Coalition Pest Monitoring Protocol

When placing pest trapping monitors it is important to remember a few things:

- Monitors should be re-locatable. Note the number and rough location of the traps in each room in case someone else has to retrieve them.
- They should be out of the way of people and the activities of the building occupants.
- Number and date all traps.
- Monitor locations should cover the site well. Use too many as opposed to too few.
- Pest Vulnerable Areas (PVAs) should always have traps present.
- Place traps near to persistent Pest Conducive Conditions (PCCs), it's always helpful to be able to demonstrate the effects of PCCs.
- Place monitors in reported hot spots.
- Treat the school like it's your Mother's home.

It's a sign of good house keeping when monitors are in place. It you use monitors to review a possible problem in a classroom. Make sure that the students and teacher understand the monitors are there to help in making sure there is no pest problem. It's a classroom, do a little teaching yourself.

PVAs

1. Kitchen/Cafeteria
   - Dry storage, dishwasher, pantry, backdoor and external cafeteria doors, floor drains, within the lower panels of serving counters.
2. Staff lounge
   - Behind vending machines, behind microwave, next to refrigerator. Remember Teachers are generally.
3. Custodian's closet
   - Under shelving, near to floor sink, external door (if present).
4. Reported Hot Zones
   - Reported in person or on Pest Monitoring Logs.
5. Special Education/kindergarten Classrooms
6. Home Economics Classrooms
7. Under/behind stage areas
8. Locker areas
9. Commissary buildings
10. Classrooms with animals/plants
11. Cluttered classrooms
12. Bathrooms
    - External doors, near cracks and crevices, near utility pipes without escutcheon plates.

Other useful places include:

Nurse's office, front offices (if they are amenable, have a pest problem, or external doors presenting problems). School nursing staff are generally interested and helpful. Front office folks can be incredibly interested and often relay reported pest sightings.

General Information:

Generally traps are placed on the floor against walls and/or on window ledges. Don't forget to check-out the naturally occurring insect traps in buildings (window ledges, floor drains, light coverings, spider webbing, etc.).

C. IPM IN SCHOOLS, MONROE MODEL Inspection Checklist

(As modified from Gouge, Schmeits, and Snyder Audit Checklist)

1. School name & district:

2. Audit Participants:

3. School site details (names, phone numbers and/or e-mails)**:**
- Age of School:
- Principal:
- Number of students:
- Area:
- Director of Operations:
- IPM Specialist:
- Grounds Supervisor:
- Building Manager:
- Number of custodians:
- Contractual custodians:
- Kitchen manager:
- School nurse:
- On-site food prep.:
- Pest Management Company:
- Waste Management:
- Perceived pests:
- Observed pests:
- Pesticide use:
- Baits:
- Monitor traps:
- Pest sighting logs:
- Training programs:
- Pest management education:
- Information systems:
- Sanitation:
- Pest Press:

1. Building Exterior

Areas to inspect:

☐ Windows & screens	☐ Dumpsters	☐ Trash cans	☐ Food areas & tables
☐ Trees & shrubbery	☐ Turf	☐ Covered areas	☐ Eves & walls
☐ Lights	☐ Conduits	☐ Cold seems	☐

i.e., are there gaps between window or screen and frame? Are dumpsters located away from building, closed, and relatively clean? Are trees overhanging building? Are shrubs shoulder-width away from building? Is there evidence of water damage on eves or walls, or spider webbing? Do lights have webbing or evidence of bird activity around them? Do they flood irrigate& does the water tend pool anywhere?

2. Kitchen

Areas to inspect:

☐ Pantry	☐ Under counters & appliances	☐ Trash cans	☐ Stored food bins
☐ Dishwashing area	☐ Floor drains & sinks	☐ Cookware storage area	☐ Garbage disposals
☐ Ceiling tiles	☐ Backdoor & exterior cafeteria doors	☐ Counter tops	☐ Pantry shelving

What to look for: Behind bulletin boards, on window sills, how close is dumpster to back door, efficiency of air-curtains on doors, external door seals, drains have metal baskets, corner clean, are floors steam cleaned or power washed periodically? Pest monitoring log available?

3. Custodian's closet – room # _____

Areas to inspect:

☐ Mops & brooms clean?	☐ Clutter?	☐ Sink	☐ Pesticides?
☐ Clutter?	☐ Racks used for brooms and mops?	☐ Shelving?	☐

4. Classrooms & nurse's office
name/room # _____

Areas to inspect:

☐ Inside cupboards	☐ Under sinks	☐ Under & behind furniture	☐ Overhead lights
☐ Teacher's cupboards	☐ Drains	☐ Corners	☐

5. Teacher's lounge ☠

Areas to inspect:

☐ Under furniture & cushions	☐ Sinks	☐ Under & behind vending machines	☐ Overhead lights
☐ Cupboards	☐ Microwave	☐ Oven	☐ Refrigerator
☐ Counters	☐ Biohazard suits needed?	☐	☐

6. Hallways, main office

name/room # _____

Areas to inspect:

□ Corners	□ Overhead lighting	□ Under & behind furniture	□ Exterior doors
□ General sanitation	□ Ventilation	□ Windows	□ Ceiling tiles
□ Bulletin boards	□	□	□

D. MEMORANDUM OF UNDERSTANDING

For the Implementation of a Pilot IPM Program into the Kyrene
School District

PRINCIPLES
I. Pesticide Environmental Stewardship Program (PESP) Partnership
Dr. Marc Lame-Indiana University, School of Public and Environmental
Affairs
John Carter-Monroe County Community School Corporation (MCCSC)
Planning Director and Grant Administrator
Jerry Jochim-MCCSC IPM Coordinator
Dr. Bobby Corrigan-RMC Pest Management
Mark Rumph, School IPM Coordinator, Auburn University Extension

II. Arizona Partners
Mary Grisier, USEPA Region 9
Dr. Paul Baker, Arizona University Extension Entomologist
David Broadstreet, Arizona Structural Pest Control Board
Stan Peterson, Director of Facilities, Kyrene School District
Mike Lindsey, PCO (Onsite Technical IPM Coordinator)

      **This program is dependent on the coordinated approach of
different entities to assure successful implementation. While this
document is not meant to be legally binding, it is, as a matter of
ethical communication, requested that each participant agree to the
following objectives and designated activities:**

OBJECTIVES
To provide education through training, demonstrate technological and program
planning innovations, develop and disseminate outreach materials, conduct
audits of pesticide use, cost and exposure outlining tangible progress for the
mitigation of risk to the school community, and is designed to be transferable to
other school communities. These objectives will be accomplished through:
    EDUCATION:
- Train change agents in Arizona to assess and implement public school IPM
  programs
- Train staff at three pilot schools in the Kyrene School District to

incorporate IPM into their existing operational activities (sanitation, maintenance, food service, health, and education)

- Train those providing pest control technology (pest monitoring and pesticide application) with the state of the art regarding child sensitive facilities

DEMONSTRATION:
- Demonstrate IPM program planning, implementation and assessment to State Lead Agencies and school districts in Arizona through the successful implementation of the IPM pilot program

OUTREACH:
- Disseminate and/or develop IPM materials to change agents in Arizona
- Disseminate and/or develop IPM materials to representative school districts in Arizona
- Assist the pilot school district in becoming future Partners in the Pesticide Environmental Stewardship Program (PESP)

RISK REDUCTION (MEASUREMENT/MONITORING):

- Develop and conduct a pest management audits (pests, pest management technologies, number, type and exposure of pesticide applications and cost of current pest management) in the pilot schools through document research, surveys, and site monitoring.

TECHNOLOGY TRANSFER:
- Transfer the diffusion techniques employed in the MCCSC model to State Lead Agencies, and other current change agents (Auburn Extension and U. AZ Extension), and to future change agents

Designated Activities

THE PESP PARTNERSHIP WILL PROVIDE:
- Education and training with regard to school staff, state change agents and pest management personnel (consisting of one training session at program initiation and one session before program completion)
- Pilot program materials for purposes of pest monitoring, and control (excluding capital goods, and termite control)
- Conduct on site inspection/treatment for purposes of program audit and pest management (consists of three visits per pilot school in coordination with bi-weekly Onsite IPM Coordinator inspections)
- Funding support if needed for personnel OT (those staff attending training)
- Aid in the development of outreach materials for local (newsletters) and statewide (newsletters/fact sheets) use
- Press Releases and regional presentations (IF REQUESTED and agreed to

by all parties)
- Communicate bi-weekly and at request with the state program partners
- Assist state program partners with their endeavors to obtain future funding for the extension of this pilot
- "on call" status for pest complaints or emergencies

THE SCHOOL DISTRICT WILL PROVIDE:
- Access to previous records related to pest management and pesticide use
- Access to three schools for inspection and pest management
- Access to personnel in those schools (mostly staff vs. teachers) for training and determination of pest problems
- Assurance that current PCOs be prohibited from treating any of the pilot schools without justification and/or communication with our team (though we welcome their participation in our training!!)
- Allow the distribution of IPM materials (newsletters) to teachers, admin and staff
- Agree to visitation by school administrators from other states (after all we are doing a national model)
- Become a PESP partner upon successful completion of the pilot program

THE STATE LEAD AGENCY AND/OR COOPERATIVE EXTENSION REPRESENTATIVE WILL PROVIDE:
- Onsite coordination and communication with regard to information dissemination in your program area
- Data gathering/sharing with regard to existing or ongoing economic and pest surveys regarding pest management in schools
- Willingness to coordinate activities with other states (dependent on travel funding)
- Tailor this program to their state, however within the confines of the MCCSC model IPM parameters
- Bi-monthly communication with a PESP Partnership representative
- Attendance and participation in at least one training session and one onsite inspection

THE ONSITE IPM TECHNICAL COORDINATOR WILL PROVIDE:
- Bi-weekly inspections (with documentation) of each pilot school for the duration of the program
- Attend all training sessions
- Attend all school technical inspections conducted by the PESP Partner
- Education to the school personnel with regard to pests, pest prevention and program status during each scheduled visit
- "on call" status for pest complaints or emergencies
- Willingness to coordinate activities with other states (dependent on travel funding)

Signatures To the Memorandum of Understanding....

Pests of the Month

MICE and ANTS

Information in this newsletter was taken directly from the School IPM Website maintained by the University of Florida Entomology and Nematology Department. Please visit this site at:
http://schoolipmifas.ufl.edu/
This site offers an excellent tutorial on head lice, which is available from your school nurse/health aide.

INSIDE THIS ISSUE

1   Mice – Biology and Control Methods

1   Website with further information

2   MCCSC IPM Coordinator

Featured Pest: MICE!
(from information provided by Dr. Robert Corrigan)

The house mouse, *Mus musculus*, meaning "little thief", is one of the most common small mammals throughout Indiana. They commonly invade schools throughout the year, but especially during the cold weather months. Although mice are not a major health threat, the potential for transmission of bacteria from their waste products always exists. Moreover, mice will gnaw on wires in offices, computer rooms, or in various electric components, causing electrical outages or short circuits.

One of the safest and most effective methods of controlling minor infestations of mice in schools or at home is the ordinary mouse snap trap. Some good bait ideas are peanut butter, bacon, nuts, raisins, popcorn, or cloth, which mice use for nests. Baits are more effective when they are tied to the trigger, and when the traps are placed perpendicular to the wall, with the trigger next to the wall. Make sure traps are placed firmly in high-activity areas for mice -- in dark corners or behind objects -- which can usually be identified if there are mouse droppings nearby. Monitor and keep traps clean, making sure to reset successful traps. Mice can be controlled without relying on poisons!

Live-catch traps are another method of controlling mice, but most mice can only survive in such traps for a few hours before succumbing to death due to stress and exposure. Cats, another famous mouse- control method, are actually less effective than you might think: they generally have no need to actively hunt mice. Finally, ultrasonic devices, which have become popular recently, have not been shown to control rodents.

For some ideas on how to prevent mouse problems in the first place, see the IPM tip box below.

Key Points for Keeping Mice Out of Schools and Homes

◊   Have all openings that allow mice to enter repaired or caulked -- this includes openings as

continued on page 2

continued from page 1

small as a dime!

◊ Remove, or have removed debris indoors and outdoors that could harbor mice, such as wood piles near foundations, clutter, or mulch piles.

◊ Have high weeds growing nearby cleared away -- weeds (and weed seeds) serve as a source of food and shelter for mice living on the outside of buildings during the warm weather months.

Keep food scraps cleaned up and store all foods so that mice do not have easy access to them. All pet foods and bird seed in classrooms (or elsewhere) should be stored off the floor and in mouse-proof containers.

ANTS

Ants become pests when they invade buildings in search of food or shelter. It is often very difficult and laborious to eliminate most ants from their outside habitat, therefore management should be targeted at preventing ants from invading structures. Unfortunately, prevention is not always successful and control actions must be implemented.

Although ants are often regarded as pestiferous, it should be noted that ants are beneficial in several ways. First, ants are predators of numerous pest insects, including fly larvae and termites. Secondly, ants aerate soil and recycle dead animal and vegetable material thus aiding in the formation of top soil. Additionally, ants are responsible for pollinating plants in some areas. Ants provide a great service to the environment, and management efforts that prevent or control ants are preferred over practices that aim to eliminate ants.

Identification and Biology

Ants are social insects that live in colonies whose members are divided into three castes: workers, queens, males. The responsibilities of the worker caste are to enlarge and repair the nest, forage for food, care for the young and queen, and defend the colony. The queen's primary duties are egg laying and directing the activities of the colony while males serve only to mate with the queens.

Ants pass through four stages of development: egg, larva, pupa, and adult. After mating with males, queens lay eggs that hatch into blind, legless larvae. The larvae are fed and cared for by worker ants. At the end of the larval stage they turn into pupae which do not feed. After a short period of time, adult ants emerge from their pupal stage and become worker ants.

The first step in management of pest ants is proper identification. Since there are many types of ants that may invade a structure it is important to identify the type of ant because most ants differ in their habits and food preferences. See Identifying Ants and Common House-Invading Ant Species.

The University of Florida offers a poster that combines line drawings, color and scanning electron microscope photographs in an identification key to help individuals identify the most common structure-invading ants.

Detection and Monitoring

Visual inspection is the most useful monitoring technique for detecting ants and can be very useful in preventing a developing infestation. A thorough inspection and prevention program is required to locate the ant source.

• Constructing a map of the school on which you can note problem areas and areas needing repair.

• A bright flashlight is mandatory. Kneepads and a mirror are helpful.

• A sealant such as outdoor caulk can be used to seal holes and cracks that ants could use to gain entry to the structure.

• Keep accurate records during the monitoring program to help formulate an IPM plan and evaluate its effectiveness.

• Careful attention should be paid to indoor areas such as kitchens and food preparation areas.

• An ant infestation may indicate that there has been a change in the methods of storing food or food waste that allows increased food sources for ants. Note how food and food wastes are stored in the area, and whether refuse containers are emptied and cleaned regularly. Inspect recycling bins to ensure that recyclables have been cleaned before storage.

• Interact with kitchen staff and custodians to learn more about the problem from their perspective.

• Ants can be attracted to snacks kept in classrooms or teachers break rooms as well as to sweet drinks accidentally spilled on the floor.

Questions about the IPM Program in the CCSD may be directed to:
Jerry Jochim
IPM Coordinator
Service Building
560 E. Miller Dr.
330-7720
jjochim@mccsc.edu

THE PEST PRESS 2

Index

Entomological Society of America, 53, 54, 211
Environmental justice, 140

F

Federal Insecticide, Fungicide, Rodenticide Act, 12, 120
Feldman, Jay, x, 42
Feral cats, 105, 126
Firebrat, 128, 182
Flea, 142
Flies, 15, 35, 89, 99, 105, 115, 116, 124, 142, 196
　Fruit, 89, 105, 116
　House, 15, 142
　Mosquito, 4, 5, 110
　Moth, 56
　Punkie, 128
　Screw Worm, 14
Fournier, Al, 48
Fox, Ed, x

G

Garnett, James, 76
Gibb, Tim, 48, 57, 87, 158
Godec, John, 192
Goldman, Lynn, 53
Golson, Nancy, 118
Gouge, Dawn, ix, 48, 99, 144, 152, 167, 181, 183, 190
Graham, Fudd, ix, 44, 48, 113, 181
Green, Tom, x, 41, 46, 202
Greene, Al, x

H

Hantavirus, 139, 141, 145
Harborage, 23, 25, 31, 104, 128, 149, 150, 182
Hawkins, Lyn, ix, 123, 129, 132, 181
Hokanson, David, x, 84
Hometown Proposal, 166
Hopi, 141, 151, 152

I

Improving Kids Environment, 41, 188
Indiana Department of Environmental Management, 91, 241
Indiana Pesticide Review Board, 201, 202, 211
Indian house cricket, 15, 99, 105, 126
IPM Institute of North America, 202

J

Jackson, Richard, 53
James, Allen, 52, 58, 209
Jochim, Jerry, ix, 43, 61, 90, 113, 121, 144, 177, 181, 186, 227
Johnson, Stephen, 53

K

Kingdon, James, 194, 197, 198, 199, 211
Kubista-Hovis, Kristi, x
Kyrene School District, 61, 100, 109, 110, 111, 128, 136, 227

L

Landrigan, Philip, 53
Langston, David, 15
Lindsey, Mike, ix, 43, 99, 106, 109, 110, 144, 175, 181, 182, 227
Luckmann, William, 6, 8, 74, 212, 220
Lumpkin, Richard, ix, 44, 114

M

Malaria, 5
Martin, Carl, ix, 47, 62, 99, 106, 144, 145, 148, 152, 181, 207
McBride, Debbie, 146
Mechanical control, 20, 29, 110, 124, 150, 191, 206, 220
Mehring, Rodney, 123
Mellencamp, John, 13
Metcalf, Robert, 6, 8, 74, 212, 220

Swain, Larry, 47, 62

ABOUT THE AUTHOR

Dr. Lame is on the faculty of Indiana University's School of Public and Environmental Affairs in Bloomington where he teaches "Environmental Management", "Management Communication", "Environmental Policy" and "Insects and the Environment". He readily assists the USEPA, non-profit children's environmental health advocate organizations with the coordination of IPM programs in schools.

Marc spent nine years of his career as an Extension IPM Specialist with the University of Arizona, Entomology Department where he was responsible for the implementation of Integrated Pest Management in cotton, and other field crops. Prior to coming to Indiana, he was a senior administrator for the Arizona Department of Environment Quality where he acted as liaison to the regulated public (industry, municipalities, and state and federal agencies), Native American tribes and environmental groups. Dr. Lame currently serves on The Indiana Department of Environmental Management's Air Toxics and Asthma Advisory Council, is on the Board of Directors for the Improving Kids' Environment Coalition (IKE), and on the Board of Directors for the International Urban Integrated Pest Management Association.

Marc thrives in Bloomington, Indiana with his wife, twin daughters and Newfoundland dogs. He considers himself an outdoorsman, naturalist and martial artist. He lives by the motto: "it is more fun to rock the boat when you are already wet".

Printed in the United States
31776LVS00006B/58-336